RussaYog

Harness Your Inner Strength
with Rope-Based Yoga

Your visit warms our hearts.

ਜੀ ਆਇਆਂ ਨੂੰ

jee aaiyaa noo

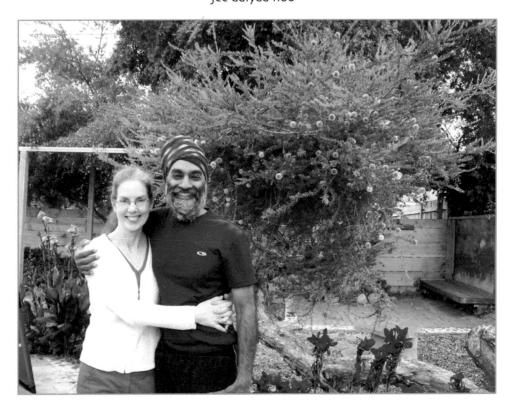

RussaYog:
Harness Your Inner Strength with Rope-Based Yoga

Jasprit Singh
Co-owner, RussaYog Yoga Studios
Professor of Applied Physics and
Electrical Engineering and
Computer Science
University of Michigan
Ann Arbor

Teresa Singh
Design and production
Co-owner: RussaYog Yoga Studios

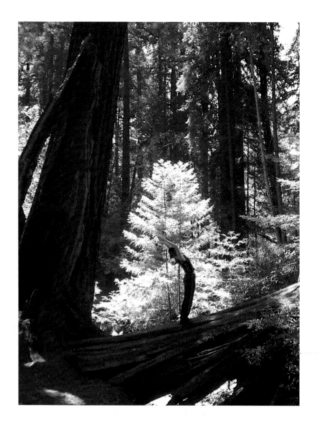

Printed by Bookmasters, Inc.
30 Amberwood Parkway
P.O. Box 388
Ashland, OH 44805

Library of Congress Cataloging-in-Publication Data
Singh, Jasprit.
RussaYog: Harness Your Inner Strength with Rope-Based Yoga/Jasprit and Teresa Singh—1st ed.

ISBN: 0-9660942-4-7
1. Authors—Non-fiction 2. Yoga—Non-fiction.
3. Fitness—Non-fiction 4. Health and Wellness—Non-fiction.

About Us

Jasprit Singh was born in New Delhi, India, in 1953. He learned holistic living from his parents and their friends. Physical abhyas (exercises), massages, meditation and kirtan (singing hymns) were integrated into daily life. After obtaining a Master's degree in Physics from Delhi University, Jasprit attended the University of Chicago where he earned a Ph.D. in Physics in 1980. He researched topics in materials and devices for information and energy conversion while working at the University of Southern California, the University of Tokyo, the Air Force Labs in Dayton, and at the University of California at Santa Barbara. His home base has been the University of Michigan, Ann Arbor, since 1985. In addition to publishing ten textbooks in areas of applied physics, electronics, and optical devices, he has published over 300 technical papers and graduated 17 Ph.D. students.

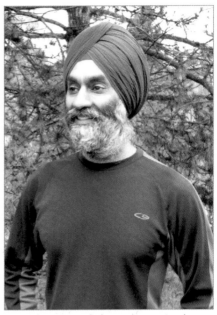
photograph by Teresa Singh

The holistic lifestyle embodied in yoga in general and RussaYog in particular has been part of Jasprit's lifestyle since childhood. He has developed the RussaYog approach over the last 40 years.
The book presented here is a synthesis of these decades of practice and teaching.

Teresa Singh was born in Illinois to parents who were involved in hosting international exchange students and families to foster intercultural understanding. Her early exposure to welcoming persons of all faiths, classes, and cultures developed in her a universal outlook on life. As a teen, Teresa was introduced to yoga and meditation and learned an appreciation of the power of the mind to guide oneself to inner peace and well-being. She continued her studies in the field of human behavior, earning a Master's degree in Social Work and an MA in Public Administration from the University of Southern California. Teresa's many years of experience working in the mental health field have given her an appreciation of the importance of meeting each challenge in life with a positive attitude.

She started teaching RussaYog in 2004 when she and her husband opened the first studio in Ann Arbor.

Jasprit and Teresa have been married since 1979 and have two sons.

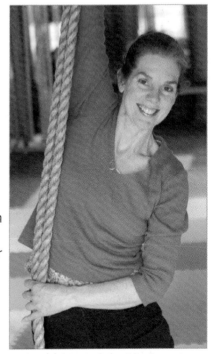
photograph by Lin Jones

RussaYog Yatra (Journey)

If you visit a large bookstore and seek out the "Health and Fitness" section you may scan dozens of books on yoga, Pilates, weight training, etc. Each style offers its own unique benefits. The yoga books contain postures developed thousands of years ago in India. Each author presents his or her own interpretation and performance style of these classical asans (poses). The reader is encouraged to learn from these books. The moment you open this book you will see it is unlike any of the books in the "Health and Fitness" aisle.

The russa (rope), anchored or free flowing, expands your dimensions. It allows you to balance, stretch, and strengthen—all with confidence. It encourages you to do movements you cannot do otherwise—thus bringing you new experiences. This book introduces you to the concept of using Mudra, Asan, and Vishram in order to success-fully approach life's challenges. Asans are not made more demanding through difficult contortions—there is no need for that. A beginner does the same asan a bit tentatively; an experienced student with alert-abandon. RussaYog movements can, at one instance, make you feel powerful like a bull; next, delicate like a butterfly. One may feel playful like a kitten at one point; and poised like a hummingbird the next. You may be flying one moment; riding a horse the next. It is up to you to enjoy the experience!

Table of Contents

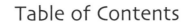

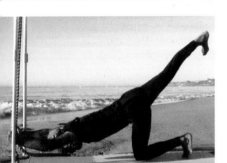

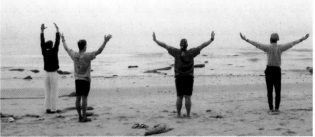

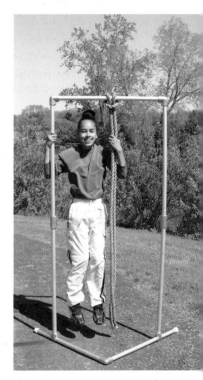

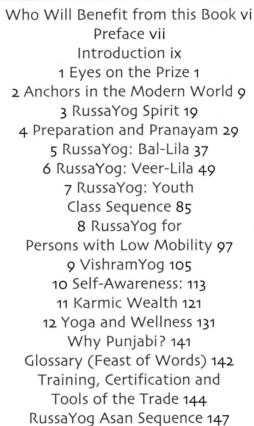

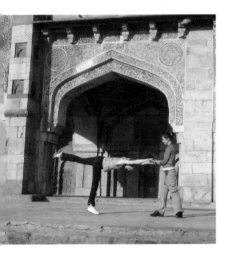

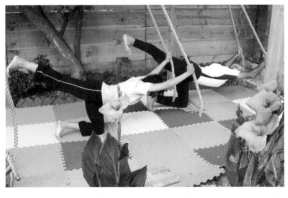

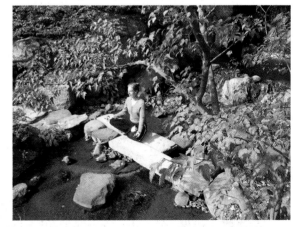

Who Will Benefit from This Book

Yoga Students: No matter what your style of yoga, you will deepen your awareness of yogic principles and their use in daily life. You will also learn a powerful style of yoga practice using ropes.

Athletes: RussaYog will complete your sport and bring balance into your body. This is an easy-to-learn yoga style centered around strength, balance, and flexibility. It will also enhance your focus and self-awareness and help prevent injuries.

Persons with low mobility: Open yourself to new possibilities.

Physical Education Teachers: Bring a fun, new approach to yoga to your students!

Yoga Teachers, Personal Trainers, Martial Arts Sensei, Dance Instructors: Incorporate new, challenging sequences into your training—also get certified in this new, powerful style of mind-body fitness.

Physical therapists, Home Health Professionals: Bring a new, adaptive style of fitness exercises to your clients.

Contact talk@russayog.com for more details about RussaYog, the Primal Shakti Yoga Trees, Retreats, and Teacher Certification.

Acknowledgements

What does it take to try something new? Trust. Curiosity. Boldness.
Thanks to all of our RussaYogis who have shared our yatra over the years.
And thanks to those who became our "models!"

the youth:
Nihal, Nirala, Ajay, Audrey, Bailey, Colleen, Isabel, Jack, Kate, Katie, Lauren, Mattie, Patrick, Quentin, Ruby, Steven.

the warriors:
Jasprit and Teresa Singh, plus: Jason Blackman, Michael Foster, Patrick Galoustian, Daljit Singh Gill, Rhonda Gilpin, Gursharan Kaur, Brian A. Kirk, Jr., Gia Massaniso Kirk, Linda Liechty, Aurora Losapio, Phil Lovalenti, Arnie Schindhaus, LaKisha Simmons, Yannick Smits, Bob Snyder, Casey Stark, Susan Todoroff, and Aurelia Webb.

and thank you to our parents:
Gurcharn Singh, Gursharan Kaur, Francis Sterling Murphy, Margaret Murphy

> In acceptance, in coherence;
> Achieve True freedom.
> As in joy, so in sorrow;
> Always in harmony, never in woe.
> As is gold, so is dust;
> As are delicacies, so are scraps.
> As is honor, so is dishonor;
> As are the mighty, so are the lowly.
> Find the path of resonance
> and become Truly free.
>
> -A description of the enlightened being by Guru Granth Sahib

PREFACE

By the time I turned five, my father, Gurcharn Singh, was bringing me along on his morning sojourn. He woke me up at 5 a.m., massaged my legs with a little mustard oil, and took me down the yet dark Delhi streets, singing shabads (hymns) when I took a pause from my questions. We strolled through parks and, as I played about, he sang and chanted, did breathwork, his asans, and various vigorous exercises. He showed me how joyful the process of physical-mental fitness is. The RussaYog fitness program presented in this book is inspired by what I observed as a child. It strives to combine the spontaneity of childhood, the commitment of adulthood, and the calmness of the age of grey hair.

The quotations in this book written in Gurmukhi script, with meanings, are words that I heard as I was growing up. They have provided me solace and I hope they benefit the readers as well.

As a child I was always fascinated by ropes. There was a beautiful Jamun tree in our courtyard and I spent several hours each day on the tree, observing life from above and using a rope to experience what a bird might feel. Or I would pretend to be powerful like the monkey god Hanuman of Ramayana, swinging around the tree.

Russas, or ropes, are intriguing entities. They bend and contort, but are incredibly strong. They immediately bring out the child in you. An older person feels young holding a rope, stretching and swaying, releasing stiffness and remembering youthful times. Is not the attraction of the Golden Gate Bridge of San Francisco due to its ropes (cables) that hold the massive structure with such grace and elegance?

I have spent most of my career as a physicist studying new materials and designing high-performance lasers and transistors at centers of innovation, like the University of Michigan, the University of Tokyo, and the University of California at Santa Barbara. Studying yoga (first from my father, then from yogis in India, and onto developing RussaYog over the last several decades) is as exciting, or perhaps more exciting, than developing a 50 gigabit laser. Having lived equal time in India, with its focus on looking inward for happiness, and in the West, with its focus on looking outward for happiness, I think it was inevitable that RussaYog would arise. I have always wanted to develop an east-west mind-body experience which is easy to learn, produces a sensuous, muscular body, and a calm-alert mind.

The RussaYog session and underlying concepts described in this book have the following goals, in addition to building a beautiful physique.

• Take yourself outside your comfort zone into a stressful (but not painful) state and deal with it with a positive attitude.

• Take your mind through the four stages of:
    Shant (calm)
    Chanchal (playful)
    Sthir (focused commitment) and
    Supt (rest)

• Make yourself aware that your inner strength is greater than you realize and allow yourself to learn how to tap into this strength.

• Develop a reflective mind that can guide you to expand your karmic wealth. Karmic wealth may include your obvious material wealth, but also extends over all life experiences. It is essential that we value our karmic wealth and perform karmas (actions) to nourish it. This idea of karmic wealth is elaborated upon in Chapter 11.

This book is the outcome of close collaboration with Teresa Singh, who is responsible not only for the artwork and design, but also the presentation of the main concepts.

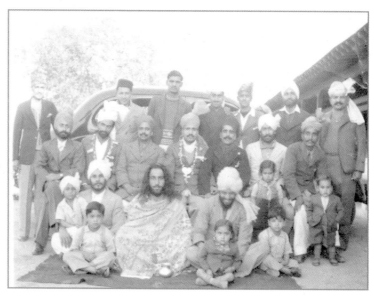

As a young man, Gurcharn Singh, Jasprit's father, travelled across India, Pakistan and Afganistan with a number of Yogi groups learning and developing his own style. Here he is (standing second from right) with a group in Pathankot, India, in January of 1939.

INTRODUCTION

Human beings have complex, four-dimensional forms—all of which need nurturing and growth. Yog or union (or yoke) symbolizes coherence between thought and action that allows such nurturing growth to occur. Desirable attributes of each of our four dimensions are:

Four Dimensions of Human Entity			
Physical	Mental	Social	Spiritual
speed	intelligence	empathy	"beyond self"view
strength	creativity	commitment	beyond "me-you"duality
flexibility	connectivity	bonding	

To achieve these attributes humans have to subject themselves to stress. Athletes, students, social reformers, and saints all have to go beyond their comfort zone to grow. Stress can produce negative outcomes, such as panic, anger, and loss of control...or positive outcomes, such as gratitude, pleasure, and positive challenge. Whether our response to a given stress is negative or positive depends upon our attitude, which is dependent upon our state of mind and our understanding of truth.

East-West Approach to Truth

The phrase "East is East and West is West and never the twain shall meet"[1] is catchy, and may have been valid a generation or two ago. Today, however, there is a greater interaction between the Eastern and Western approaches to life. Globalization, environmental concerns, recognition that the Earth needs to be treated with respect...are all making East and West more respectful of each other. Nowhere is this more apparent than in health care. The West has recognized that the human body is more than biology and chemistry. The East has recognized the benefit of the scientific method.

When you travel to a historic "holy site" in Europe and in India, you can experience the stereotypical differences between East and West, described here:

West	East
• preference for order	• comfortable in chaos
• alter "natural conditions" to suit human desires	• Alter human desire to suit "natural conditions"
• encourage individual development	• encourage loss of ego
• find truth through scientific analysis ...very useful in the physical world.	• find truth through meditation and intuition...very useful for human consciousness and happiness

[1]Rudayrd Kipling, "The Ballad of East and West"

The different approaches to life are also reflected in personal health and mind-body development. In the West, one may learn about the details of muscles, bones, and organs, and the uses of drugs and medicines, whereas in the East the focus is on the "feeling" created by balance and good karma. This is reflected by Ashtanga, the eight limbs of yoga used to define human experiences, briefly summarized here.

1. Yama, or rules of social behavior: Includes being honest, generous, etc.
2. Niyama, or disciplined living: Related to individual daily habits.
3. Asana: Establishing a mind-body awareness. This is what we generally speak of when we refer to "yoga."
4. Pranayama: Usage of breath as life force.
5. Pratyahara: Opening the inward-looking eye.
6. Dharana: Bringing your desires in harmony with the natural state.
7. Dhyana: Focused awareness where nothing distracts you.
8. Samadhi: Merging into the infinite where any state is acceptable.

The term yoga is now usually used for the third branch (Asana). This branch of yoga is based on a number of tools designed to focus and harness the power of the mind and body. These include:

1. Drishti, or sight: Focusing both the outer and the inner eye can suppress the mind's drifting nature.
2. Pranayama, or breathwork: One of the more powerful ways to harness the mind. Focused breathwork including rhythmic breathing, is well known to focus the mind.
3. Chanting: Especially in a group chanting can take the mind into a coherent zone.
4. Performing asans, or difficult body postures, focus the mind.
5. Mudras, or unusual expressions of the hands, fingers, face, eyes, and tongue: focuses the mind.
6. Fasting: Can clear the mind of cobwebs.
7. Drugs: Can offer the user a temporarily sharp, focused mind—although at considerable penalty.

Yoga, familiar to most, has used Drishti, Pranayama, and Asans to harness the mind-body connection to create balance and well-being. The RussaYog session described in this book allows the yogi to take his/her mind-state from calm to dithering to focused to restful. All four mind-states are critical for growth as described in the book. The ultimate growth is spiritual where we see ourselves in all creation and experience a true sense of freedom.

An additional contribution to the understanding of the human mind-body dimension is through the description of chakras (circles) which describe various layers of human complexity. Each of these chakras need to be developed in order to reach enlightenment. Chakras are briefly described next, along with their physical location. The interested reader may find books that also describe specific planets, colors, gemstones, animal properties, scents, etc., that are associated with the chakras. We will not elaborate upon these here.

CHAKRAS OF
HUMAN MIND-BODY DIMENSION

1. Mooldhara:
Root supports centered in the
adrenal glands (base of the spine)
2. Svadhisthana:
Creative force centered in
reproductive organs
3. Manipura:
Energy source in the pancreas
(navel to solar plexus)
4. Anahata:
Heart, associated with the thymus
5. Visudha:
Expression, located in the thyroid
6. Ajna:
Intuition (third eye), pituitary gland
7. Sahasrara:
Consciousness, pineal gland

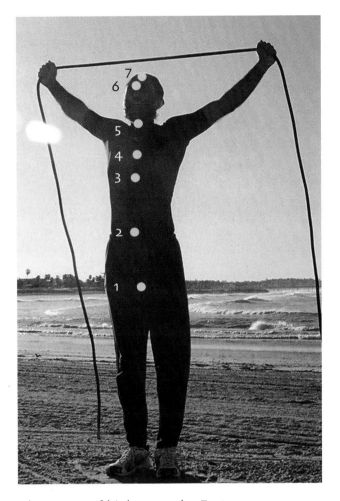

Regardless of whether you use the Western language of biology or the Eastern language of feeling, when you feel good, you know it, provided you are in tune with yourself. In this book, you will experience and enjoy—with minimal discourse. The best approach to reach human happiness should synthesize the best of the West and the best of the East. This is the basis of the RussaYog approach—it is both empirical and meditative-intuitive. It does not condone blind acceptance, nor does it support the idea that analytical techniques can fathom all of the complexities of human consciousness.

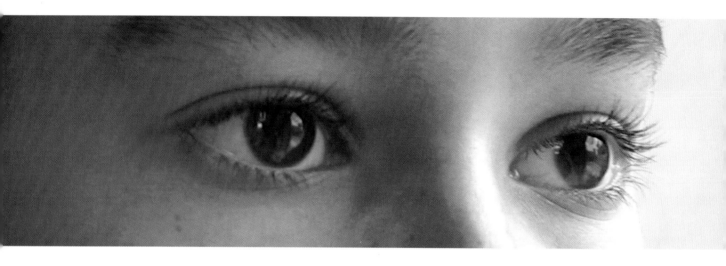

The only chain that a man can stand

Is that chain o' hand in hand

Keep your eyes on the prize, hold on...

"Keep Your Eyes on the Prize," folk song by Alice Wine 1956
adapted from early 20th century American hymn "Gospel Plow"
(also "Eyes on the Prize:" PBS documentary on the American Civil Rights Experience)

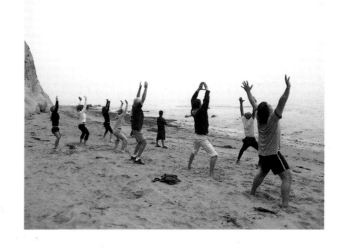

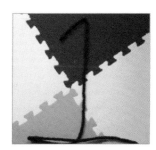

EYES ON THE PRIZE

What is the prize we want in life? We each want the freedom to grow—into our glorious potential. We want to grow into healthy, strong human beings, unafraid, strong of limb, with lustrous hair, erect posture. We want to expand our mind—to be intelligent with bright, shining eyes marvelling at and learning from Nature's school. We want to grow socially—with nurturing and warm friends and an accepting society. Most importantly, we want to grow spiritually—to love all beings of this beautiful world. We want to see ourselves in others—to find love and to give love.

If we so desire to have freedom to grow—just as a sapling seeks sunlight and nutrients to grow into a giant redwood—what is stopping us? Bonds—real and imaginary—bind us down, stunting our growth. It is our duty to search for these bindings—some seen, some unseen—and cut them off so we can fulfill our purpose.

Bindings for Girls

The largest group of people who are still denied the freedom to grow are girls (who, of course, become women who, among other contributions, nurture families and raise societies). What are the bindings on girls? In most cultures very obvious bindings, such as foot bindings, neck-stretching bracelets, circumcision, etc., have disappeared, although some societies still suffer from them. More subtle bindings are cultural and emotional.

MYTHOLOGY-BASED BINDINGS

In many of the world's great mythologies a woman's role is often subservient or that of a seductress. Since mythologies have deep impact on the human psyche, self-imposed barriers are formed in a young child's mind.

"GOD"-GRANTED BINDINGS

Many of the world's great religious philosophies have been, unfortunately, interpreted in such a way that a woman's role is secondary to a man's or is a degrading role. While enlightened people of faith may not take religious passages literally, many believers hold on to literal interpretations.

CULTURAL BINDINGS

In many cultures young girls are supposed to "act with modesty" which often translates into no free play, no dancing, no standing tall, no laughing out loud. Then there are also cultures which entice young girls into acting overtly sexual by dressing as young women, paying enormous attention to their appearance and to what boys think of them. It may be fair to say that apart from girls growing up in some enlightened families, most girls worldwide suffer from some loss of "free" growth that would allow them to feel and nurture their own inner talents.

Caucasian Men

Now you may be shocked at this title. How could white men—the rulers of the world, the writers of history, the interpreters of God's laws—suffer from any bindings? Unfortunately, the expectations of a man's man—unemotional, rigid, ready to fight— does not make for happy social-spiritual growth. Depression, mid-life crisis, loss of love, is suffered acutely by this seemingly privileged group. White men need to undo the bindings of social expectations, historical burdens (throw away the White Man's Burden, guys) and identification with a mythical hero who does not deal well with love and emotions.

Men of Color

Well, what remains? Yes, non-white men also face their own bindings. People of color around the world face loss of ability to freely travel and explore opportunities, have poor access to education and health, and so on.

FINAL BINDING: EGO

The ultimate binding on all of us is placed by our own ego. Our ego prevents us from becoming truly universal. Me, my family, my class, my race, my country…each places its own binding. If the "me-you duality" is shattered, all other bindings disappear.

> In Ego lives the draining sickness, but in it also lies the elixir.
>
> ਹਉਮੈ ਦੀਰਘ ਰੋਗ ਹੈ ਦਾਰੂ ਭੀ ਇਸ ਮਾਹਿ
>
> Haumai deeragh rog hai daru bhi is mahi

The ultimate goal of those seeking light is reduction of arrogance. However, humility should not be confused with servitude, fear, and weakness.

Eyes on the Prize: Expanding the Boundaries

How does one tear off the bindings that prevent freedom of full growth? The first step is to understand the source of the bindings. Shackles that limit our physical development include: too little food, too much food, lack of exercise, and unhealthy habits. Mental shackles arise from: superstitions, baseless fears, loss of trust due to betrayal. Social bindings come from belief in racial superiority/inferiority, gender biases, caste, creed, and wealth biases.

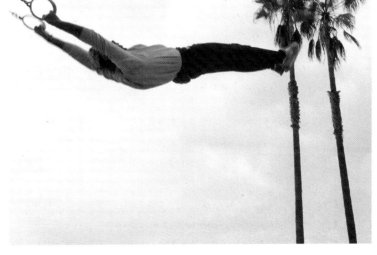

Finally, spiritual limits arise from placing dogma, not love, at the core of spirituality.

Many of our fears are deeply buried in our mind and may have been placed when we were children by strict social and cultural boundaries—or by having dysfunctional families. The process of finding these fears and dispelling them requires first understanding them and then discarding them.

To maintain focus on the prize of true freedom one needs a "coherent" approach to life where every "karma" or action pushes us toward the prize. The techniques of yogabhyas or "coherent practice" allow us to do so. Yogabhyas (the practice of yoga) is becoming increasingly important for the modern world. The approach described in this book is based on empirical evidence—do it and feel it—and not on dogma. The approach is based on a three-fold toolset comprised of: simran, or meditation, to keep the mind, calm, optimistic and focused; niyam or discipline, to ensure that life choices are consistent with our goals; and shakti or power needed for making any effort.

ਤੜੀ ਕਲਾ unbounded optimism

ਸਿਮਰਨ SIMRAN (MEDITATION)

A meditative mind is a calm-alert mind which can see the link between past, present, and future. It is needed to keep our eyes on the prize—no matter what the prize. Simple techniques can create a meditative mind. RussaYog practice as described in later chapters utilizes these techniques. They can also be practiced anywhere, anytime, using the following approach:

• Visualize highly positive experiences such as playing on the beach, being with friends, in natural beauty, etc.

• Associate a simple word or words with all these images (eg., chardi kala or unbounded optimism). Practice this association until the words fill your mind instantly with positive feelings, dissipating fears, arrogance, and worry. Thus train your mind to be optimistic, joyful, and more self-aware. Be patient with yourself and keep practicing these techniques.

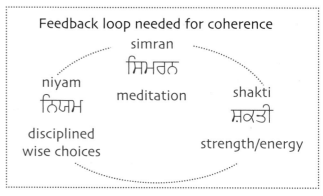

Feedback loop needed for coherence

ਨਿਯਮ NIYAM (DISCIPLINE)

No change occurs without carving out new pathways. Without discipline one falls back into the old rhythm whenever one is under stress. If you want to make an exercise program or a healthy eating program a part of your life, build it into your regular schedule. Just as you would not think of leaving home in the morning without brushing your teeth, discipline can make good practices an integral part of your day.

ਸ਼ਕਤੀ SHAKTI (POWER)

Just like a car cannot move without fuel, we cannot convert thoughts into reality without power. We need a strong body, powered by strong muscles, in addition to a strong mind, to get going.

Yogabyas as a Powerful Nourishment

The practice of yoga, and especially RussaYog described in this text, is a powerful way to harness your inner and external strength to allow growth of your mind, body, and spirit. The central spirit of RussaYog is described by ਚੜੀ ਕਲਾ—unbounded optimism.

In order to achieve your own growth and to fulfill your own talents you need to remove the fears that limit you (and decide where you do not want to go, ie., which activities are allergic and toxic to you).

To reach the state of joy and optimism we need to practice several mind-exercises. Just as we use physical exercise to build specific muscles, these mind-exercises are needed to reach the spirit of chardi kala. Just by reminding yourself of the following words, you will benefit—that's right, just continual reminders are all that are needed!

Ten Reminders

ਸ਼ਾਂਤ SHANT (CALM)

If you are in a noisy room you cannot hear things that are useful and important for you. You need to quiet your mind so you can think in peace. Modern life often makes it difficult to just be quiet for some time. The non-stop stimuli we face often from childhood brings us to a point where the shant mind is scary. But you need this state to answer, "What is it that I need and what are the paths I should take?" To reach the shant state, shut off, as much as you can, the external stimuli (TV, noise, arguments...) and also internal stimuli (worry, anger, negative self-statements...).
With depth and purpose, repeat, "Shant, shant, shant."

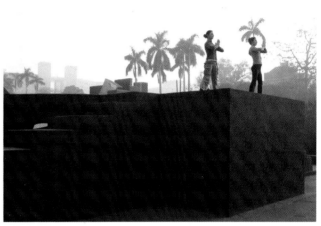

ਜਾਗਿਆ JAAGYA (AWAKE)

Our outer senses (sight, hearing, taste, touch, smell, and balance) need to awaken so we are aware of how we are interacting with the world. Also our inner sense which tell us how we are feeling, why we are doing what we are doing, need to be awake. Self-awareness in body and mind is essential to make wise choices.
Reminder: "Jaagya, jaagya, jaagya."

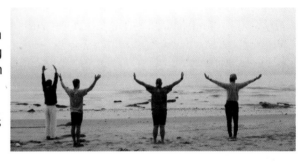

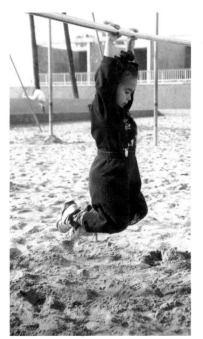

ਅਭੈ ABHAY (FEARLESS)

You need to clear your mind of fear before you can make good decisions. It is obvious that if someone uses violence to make you do something, that would not be a good choice for you. Fear of the mind is invisible, but it has the same effect—making you take paths that do not allow you to grow.
Reminder: "Abhay, Abhay, Abhay."

ਧਿਆਨ DHYAN (ATTENTIVE MIND). The mind is totally attentive and focused on the task at hand. The ancient story from Mahabharat comes to mind.

Dronacharya is training the five Pandava brothers in the art of archery
and asks each one separately to set his sight on a bird's eye.
As each one aims
before shooting the arrow,
he asks each brother what he sees.
Each of the first four brothers answers,
"The bird,
the branches nearby,
the tree,
and you, master"...
When Arjun's turn comes, he simply answers,
"The eye."
"What else, Arjun?" asks Drona.
"Only the eye."

In Dhyan the mind is constant, in the sthir state.
Reminder: "Dhyan, dhyan, dhyan."

ਅਨਹਦ ANHAD (WITHOUT BOUNDARIES).
You have to purposefully push the boundaries away. How else can you explore and grow? And with an alert, unafraid mind, you can then decide if you need the boundary or not. Not all boundaries may be bad for you.
REMINDER: "Anhad, Anhad, Anhad."

ਨਿਸ਼ਚਿੰਤ NISHCHINT (WORRY FREE). Worry is the friction of our lives. Like sand caught in a gear, or potholes on a road, worry dissipates our energies and adds little.
REMINDER: "Nishchint, Nishchint, Nishchint."

ਬਲਵਾਨ BALVAN (POWERFUL). Nothing happens without power, strength, energy. To move you need strength.
Reminder: "Balvan, Balvan, Balvan."

ਸੁੰਦਰ SUNDAR (BEAUTIFUL). It is important to believe that Nature has made a beautiful form in you. Many young people, especially (otherwise accomplished) girls, have a feeling that their appearance needs changing. Issues around eating disorders are often linked to a completely incorrect sense of one's beauty.
Reminder: "Sundar, Sundar, Sundar."

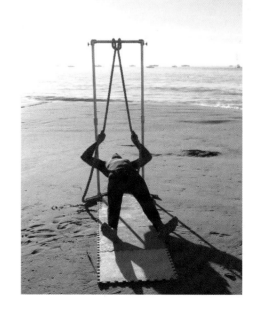

ਭਰੋਸਾ BHAROSA (TRUST).
We have all suffered some degree of betrayal. However, in order to grow we need to be trusting—of nature and of people. Of course we need to learn to avoid those who have betrayed us. In addition, can others trust us? Fulfilling a commitment is essential to build the strength and confidence needed to grow. Reminder: "Bharosa, Bharosa, Bharosa."

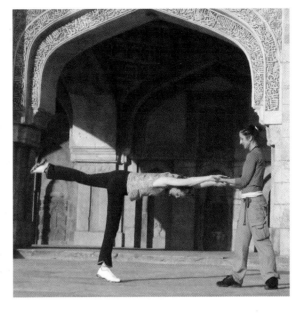

ਚੰਚਲ CHANCHAL (PLAYFULNESS).
A playful mind is needed to be able to forgive, to move on, and to explore, and enjoy new experiences.
  Reminder: "Chanchal, Chanchal, Chanchal."

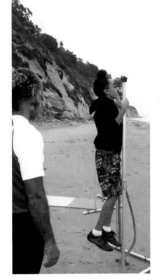

To most readers the Indian languages used here are not familiar. Why use them, instead of equivalent English words?
I feel that the use of a new sound instead of a familiar one helps you concentrate and see greater meaning in the concept it embodies. And, memorizing new words provides exercise for your brain as well!
(see the Feast of Words, page 142)

In this book we will see how one can use the RussaYog sessions to develop more fully all of these mind states.

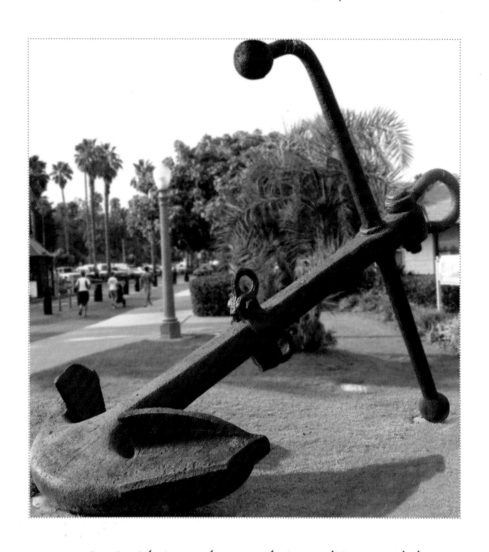

Truth, the highest virtue. Higher still, true living.

ਸਚਹੁ ਓਰੈ ਸਭੁ ਕੋ ਉਪਰਿ ਸਚੁ ਆਚਾਰੁ

Sach ourai sabh ko oupar sach aachaar

. . . .

This above all:

To thine own self be true.

And it must follow,

as the night the day,

Thou canst not then be false to any man.

-Shakespeare, in Hamlet, Act 1, Scene 3

In the modern world where lifespans are approachinng the centruy mark, can anyone afford to not have a lifelong mind-body fitness plan? Invest in yourself!

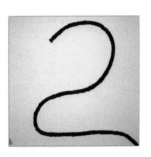

ANCHORS IN THE MODERN WORLD

How do we derive peace of mind and joy in our lives? And how do we find meaning in our lives? Clearly, material well-being is not enough to bring joy to us. According to a 2007 study by the United States Center for Disease Control (CDC), the highest number of drug prescriptions in the USA are for depression—more than prescriptions for high blood pressure, heart disease, and diabetes. Human life has always been full of strife, struggle, and sorrow, but one may argue that for most of the world's population living in developed countries, modern times with widespread access to goods and services should be a time for joy. What happened?

Our joy comes through external sources (outside ourselves) and internal sources. External sources include things that are pleasing to our senses—beautiful sights, food, music, caressing, cool breezes, and aromatic experiences. Our internal joy comes from our belief and value system—faith, participation in rituals and work and our understanding of the universal plan.

While realizing that human experience has always been stressful and often full of sorrow, the modern world offers additional sources of stresses, while alleviating others. Modern life may be characterized with an enormous access to new choices—travel, food, other ethnic experiences, sensory pleasures through technology, etc. Of course, not all of the world's population is enjoying these choices. But perhaps thirty per cent of the world population is experiencing these "modern life" choices arising from globalization, revolutions in technology, and the Civil Rights Movement (including the Women's movement).

Religions and Culture: Anchors Under Stress?

For a great part of human history religion and cultural beliefs have been a big source of comfort and solace for humanity. These have been the primary anchors for societies. However, with globalization and mass movements of people around the world as well as advances in science and women's rights, many of the obvious "truths" and practices in religions are being challenged. In its essence religion provides a connection between self and the universe. However, most religions are layered with dogma as well. Most religions begin by offering a view of the Creation of the Universe, the deeds that are the source or sorrow, and how one can redeem oneself and reach happiness.

The Creation theories of most religions have elements which contradict science and many have elements that place woman in a position of either a spoiler or a seductress. With advances in both science and women's rights believers have to find interpretations of their religion that reconcile with science and women's movements.

Is it possible to hold the Creation theories as literal truth and yet interact with people of diverse races, genders, faiths, castes, and color, in a loving, respectful way? Clearly in a democracy all people have to be treated according to their actions (karmas) in this life. How people of faith interpret their faiths is an important personal issue and a societal issue. If these issues are not resolved, religion may become an increasing source of conflict.

Bounties of Modern Life

The modern world in which most of the developed countries' population lives has enjoyed incredible abundance, thanks to science and technology, globalization, capital market forces, and the civil rights movement. These modern forces have also created massive disruptions. However, a large number of people can now enjoy (or suffer from overuse) bounties that a generation ago were only available to aristocracy and the super-rich. Theses bounties have provided new anchors for us— providing promises of comfort and solace. They have also created confusion, anxiety, and negative stress. The purpose of this book is to allow us to develop techniques and tools so we can enjoy the benefit of modern life with balance and poise.

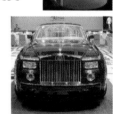

Let us examine some of the bounties which are now anchoring our lives.

FOOD

Food is one of life's great pleasures. Long after our other senses are weakened by age, we can still enjoy a delicious meal—and then enjoy some more. For most of human existence food was scarce for a great part of the year, so we are hardwired to associate food with comfort, pleasure, and security. Our body uses food so efficiently that very little is needed to stay healthy. Much has been written about how food based comfort is impacting human health. Can self-awareness and other sources of happiness replace excessive food?

CONSUMPTION OF GOODS

As with food globalization has created a flood of goods for us to sample and enjoy. And as with food we can easily go overboard. There is no denying the pleasures of consumption—a fine car, granite countertops, a Rolex watch. Consumption does create economic activity and job opportunities. But as with food, a loss of balance can force you to become a slave of the consumer society, spending your precious life paying for the goodies. In addition, the impact of consumption on Earth's health is becoming a serious issue.

MIND-ALTERING DRUGS

If the outside world is so difficult to deal with, how about altering our perception of reality? Alcohol, weed, cocaine, acid, pills...all help disconnect from whatever reality one is facing. People describe blissful (and horrible) experiences from drug trips. Unfortunately, drugs do get addictive and one can pay a terrible price for those mind trips. Even legal drugs designed to help people who genuinely need them can be easy to abuse.

TOURISM

Fifty years ago only royalty and diplomats had the pleasure of travel. Now ordinary people can travel to fascinating lands and experience unusual sounds, sights, tastes, and cultures. The personal growth that comes from travel is undeniable. However, here also one has to find balance. Travel can have impact on environment and on the local culture as well.

WORK AND CAREER

Career options have greatly expanded, especially for women and people of color. Most modern offices have people of different races, genders, and religions working in the same space. A good career where your intellect and social skills can grow is a tremen-dous source of joy. But...you can also become obsessed with work and work politics.

PLAY AND SPORTS

Athletic activity is another area where modern life has offered new possibilities. A couple of generations ago it was rare for a fifty year old to play sports. Now you can find cyclists, swimmers, soccer players, and roller bladers enjoying these sports well into "old" age. Sports creates its own elation and allows unique social bonding experiences. However, it can be a source of injuries to joints and ligaments, even as it helps the heart and lungs.

ENTERTAINMENT AND MEDIA/ARTS

A great source of pleasure is films, art, music, video games—creations of an imaginative world where one can fantasize and dream.

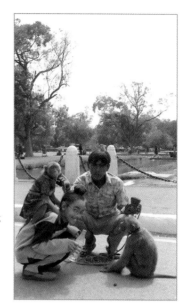

If we examine the modern offerings listed above we see that a great deal of our lives revolve around them. Without judicious use, we lose our balance and are led into an unhealthy lifestyle. Our bodies and minds have developed over thousands of years, while in just one generation, our food habits, work habits, entertainment habits, have transformed. Where once humans were preoccupied with lack of choice, now we are preoccupied with making intelligent, wise choices.

Modern Lifestyle and the Incredibly Efficient Human Body

The human body is a remarkably efficient machine. To survive the general lack of food for thousands of years (until about 50 years ago) the human machine had no choice but to be efficient. However, given the sudden abundance of food, our efficient body is causing a lot of misery—especially in prosperous societies. In fact, new kinds of diet pills, meat-based, high-protein diets, etc., are touted to reduce the human efficiency by speeding up our metabolism. It is as if everyone had an oil well in their back yard and were obligated to use up the 100 gallons per day that it spewed out!

> ...once humans were preoccupied with lack of choice, now we are preoccupied with making intelligent, wise choices.

Modern industrial life not only provides us enormous material resources (abundant food, cars, TVs, drugs...); it also magically ensnares us to spend a big chunk of our lives consuming these goodies. There are those individuals who can maintain balance and not fall into this trap. But for most people, it is difficult to step back and achieve a sense of balance—to enjoy what modern science, technology, and efficient capitalism gives us without completely exchanging our lives for material goods. A common by-product of the modern lifestyle is adverse stress (a sense of loss of control) and over-consumption.

This balancing act does not end at consumption. Additional challenges strain our physical well-being. These challenges arise from imbalanced forces that we must confront everyday to succeed in modern societies:

CHALLENGES OF MODERN LIFE

• Imbalanced position during the day: Jobs (in factories or in cubicles) require being in contorted or slouched positions for hours everyday. Without conscious choice people gradually develop aching backs. Their abdominals and shoulders slouch forward.

• Rushed food consumption: Eating, one of the most important activities, is often rushed to fit the schedule that we find ourselves in. Not only do families avoid cooking a healthy meal, the food is also gobbled down rapidly, leading to higher consumption. By simply slowing down the speed at which we put food into our bodies—giving us time to dwell on what we are doing—we can provide a balance to thought-free consumption.

• Lack of physical activity/"Bad" physical activity: Lack of physical activity has been blamed extensively in newspapers and magazines for our physical fitness dilemma. Indeed, there are few jobs which provide us the needed 8-10 miles of walking (or an equivalent) for which our bodies are designed. However, keep in mind that some of the people with very poor health are people who do physical work at their jobs. A drive through Central Valley of California shows thousands of workers bent over, picking fruits or vegetables. They certainly get a lot of exercise. But observe such a person at age fifty. His shoulders are hunched, wrists and fingers ache.
The highly imbalanced postures in which many laborers work cause them problems that are due not to inactivity, but to "bad" activity.

• Coping with the here-and-now: Perhaps the greatest challenge of modern living is the difficulty to take a broader look at how we spend our lives. After all, most of us would agree that our life and those of our loved ones are priceless. Yet we often end up exchanging it for trivial pursuits.
A day that should start with unhurried meditation starts with a cold sweat and a car stuck in rush hour. The irony is that a meditative view of our activity can greatly improve our efficiency because we can "see from afar" where we are heading.

The solution to well-being in modern life is not to become a recluse, not to abandon all social/material ties and run to the caves (although that may work for some). Rather the solution lies in finding balance and coherence in our actions and thoughts. Overall, modern life is pretty good, and for those who find balance and coherence it is really good. In fact, the balanced life that takes the best from science, technology, market forces, and mental/spiritual well-being can reach an utopian existence.

One of the great challenges of living in a market place-driven economy (ie., modern capitalism) is that we gradually learn to value only those experiences that have a price tag on them. With the exception of a few wise persons, we forget that a hug from a friend or a child, conversation with a good friend, a walk in the park with pristine views, are also valuable, even though there is no price tag attached to these experiences. If we can live with the efficiency of the market place, yet develop the meditative state needed to define our total karmic wealth as not just our bank balance, but also our well-being, friends, children, clean air, etc., we could truly be in harmony.

Karma-Fruit Relation

To reach any goal, ie., to obtain any fruit, we need to do actions or karmas. According to physics (and our own experiences) karma can be of several types:

Every fruit needs karma	
Effort	Fruit
Nutrition/Food	Health
Exercise	Strong muscles
Education	Good career
Meditation	Negative stress-free living
Shouldering responsibilities	Good long term relationships

Random or incoherent. Each subsequent action pays no attention to the previous action. In this mode very little fruit is reaped, since the actions do not reinforce each other. It is like you spend an hour in the gym working out, then have a nutritious meal, but then party all night;

Destructive. Each subsequent karma destroys the positive effects of the previous karma. There is no fruit in this sort of karma. It is as if you plant a seed, then dig it up and throw it away.

Coherent. Each karma reinforces the previous karma. In this state your goals can be reached almost effortlessly. This is the state of sthir, also called sehej (balance and coherence). Each karmic effect enhances the previous one. To fully benefit from coherent karma one needs to understand the karma-fruit relation. See Figure 1. Coherent karma is done with positive feedback from the inside and outside world. The karma-fruit relationship has four distinct regions:

1) lossy,
2) coherent,
3) saturation, and,
4) catastrophic failure.

To avoid catastrophic failure learn to broaden your horizons—develop a more Universal outlook. In the language of spirituality, it would mean lowering your sense of ego. This may involve channeling your efforts to issues beyond yourself. We would ideally like to be near the end of region II where, with little effort, we get a lot accomplished. Yogic exercises are developed to reach this state, and a meditative mind also learns to avoid the catastrophic state.

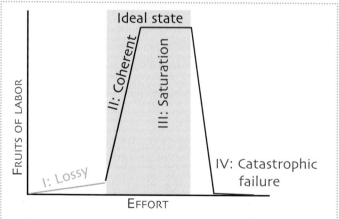

Figure 1: A general relation between effort made toward any goal and the resulting fruit. As explained in the text there is an ideal "zone" where a small extra effort produces large fruit.

I: Lossy region: Initially as effort is made there is little or no visible fruit. This is because the effort is used up just to maintain status quo. A certain minimum effort has to be made to realize the fruit.

II: Coherent state: Beyond a certain level of effort, and with the right support system, one goes into the coherent "zone" where with very little extra effort the fruit increases rapidly. Each little effort reinforces the previous one. This zone is reached when there is inner and outer feedback, which allows one to maintain coherence. Inner discipline and forces and outer environment (positive friends, positive teachers, etc.) allow us to reach this state.

III: Saturation: Eventually the fruit gets overripe, even when the effort is coherent. This is because the side effects of the fruit create negative repercussions. The side effects may be arrogance after becoming the CEO of a company, or self-absorbed state after achieving a beautiful body. The positive feedback that sustained the coherent effort starts to disappear.

IV: Catastrophic failure: If nothing is done to avoid the negative forces arising from "success," a dramatic failure occurs and the fruit disappears completely. For an athlete, excessive effort may result in torn muscles or ligaments, or a blown knee. For a businessman it may result in family disintegration or depression.

SELF-AWARENESS AND DIVERSE SOURCES OF JOY

Modern life has brought pleasures to ordinary people which, until a few decades ago, were only available to aristocracy and the super-wealthy. However, it is increasingly clear that while under consumption is a problem for humans, so is over consumption. Within a generation many parts of the world have seen populations going from mal-nourished to obese. As noted in the previous pages, the relationship between consumption and joy is not linear.

One must approach the various forms of consumption with a thoughtful, self-aware mind in order to avoid over-consumption. A self-aware mind allows one to recognize when the consumption or action needs to stop, since greed in action will bring lesser fruit. Additionally, it is important to develop multiple sources of pleasure so that one does not become dependent upon just one source. If you enjoy food, play, dance, socialization, quietness, etc., you can be mindful and switch to many sources of joy.

Creativity, Balance and Coherence: Challenges

Humans have always struggled to find balance between total immersion and total abandonment in nearly everything. We struggle to find balance between emaciation and obesity, ascetic life and gluttony, subservience and arrogance, self-hatred and snobbery, self-absorption and caring for others. We search for a healthful diet, responsible consumption, courage, and love. Yoga is the 5,000 year-old approach to provide exercises to reach this balance. Although the test of balance is real life—disease, joy, family life, social styles, etc.—yoga provides simple simulations where one can learn to achieve balance. The hope is that yogic exercises can then be carried out into real life and applied to real stress-inducing situations. Just like a flight simulator can help prepare a pilot for real life flying, yoga can serve as a stress simulator.

Prakriti (Nature) seems to have played two great jokes upon us. In order to achieve any desirable goal we need to take ourselves outside our comfort zones, i.e., place ourselves under stress. If this stress is handled positively, growth occurs. If it is handled negatively, the result is disastrous. The second great joke is that it is so difficult to build something beautiful, but very easy to degrade anything beautiful we have built. Prakriti has, however, not entirely been mean. She has also ensured that unimaginable treasures are ours to be had if we follow some simple rules of harmony and balance.

Before learning the physical aspect of the RussaYog asans (ie., postures), let us remember the five principles of balance and harmony:

1. By knowing & acting upon Truth one can attain balance and well-being.	Truth about good nutrition and exercise brings physical health. Truth in universal love brings spiritual balance. Use Truth to set your goals— whatever they may be. Use your own life guidance and other people who love you to help in your search for Truth.
2. The wealth available to us is much greater than we can ever imagine.	To realize and achieve great wealth (not just material) prepare yourself to go beyond the threshold (or beyond your comfort zone). This may require physical discipline, mental discipline, or spiritual discipline. Be willing to pay the price of crossing the threshold.
3. Keep your Karmic efforts coherent to reach your goal.	Let each action reinforce the benefits of the past action; not negate it.
4. Surround yourself with the positive energy of supportive friends and loved ones.	Also be willing to accept their support.
5. Excess physical (material), intellectual, and social growth will eventually become a liability.	Only in the spiritual sphere (love for all) can one grow indefinitely without inducing a catastrophic breakdown (discussed earlier in this chapter).

As we will see in this text, the ancient science and practice of yoga, enhanced by RussaYog techniques, allows you to gather your own diffuse and incoherent actions into a coherent, powerful state which allows you to reach your hidden strengths. Such coherent focusing does occur occasionally in our lives. It happens momentarily when a father opens the jaws of a tiger that has clasped his teeth onto his little boy's arm in a zoo; with the roar of fans in a stadium when a high jumper is suddenly able to leap 6 inches above her personal best. We all have such coherent moments—when we can uncoil our hidden energy (or kundalini as it is known in yoga). But few of us can do so on demand.

The Four Mind-States

To fully enjoy the treasures Prakriti has in store for us we need to exploit the power of our mind or man-shakti (man=mind). Four categories can be used to describe the mind's state (man avastha):

Shant (calm, at peace)	Chanchal (dithering, sampling)	Sthir (locked, focused)	Supt (sleeping, shut-off)

All four states are critical for a balanced life and it may be argued that we should spend some time each day in all four states. The RussaYog session described here will take you through all four states in about an hour.

The shant avastha is necessary to start out any endeavor. When you start in this state (rather than with anxiety, anger, grudges, etc.) it becomes easy to sort through life's fog.

To understand the chanchal and sthir mind think of the radio in your car. The chanchal state is as if your radio were in the scan mode. You jump from station to station and sample for a few seconds each offering. This is the "child-like" state where one samples one experience, then jumps to another, and so on. The chanchal state is essential for creativity, for "out-of-the-box" thinking. It is essential to choose the endeavor that is correct for you.

As you drive your car, your radio on the scan mode you suddenly encounter a station you like and you lock it in. Now you are in the sthir state. While you need to be in the chanchal state to find out what fits you, without the sthir state nothing gets accomplished. In the sthir state you are focused on your goal, and all actions work coherently to move you towards your goal. This is the state of the perfect warrior, householder, business person. This is the meditative state where almost without effort you are focused and in tune with the world. In the supt, or off, state you recover from your efforts.

We need to enjoy all four states everyday, although the relative time spent in each state may vary with life stages. Without the chanchal state we lose our sense of humor, take ourselves too seriously, and become one-dimensional. Without sthir state we are dreamers, but cannot accomplish anything. We may be the life of the party, but no one can count on us. Without the shant state, our blood pressure rises, we react to stress with panic and anger. Without supt state we are headed towards a fatigued, dry life. It is important to understand the coherent or sthir state, since this is where all growth and accomplishments occur.

In this book we will discuss tools that RussaYog uses to bring us into each of these four mind-states and allow our balanced growth.

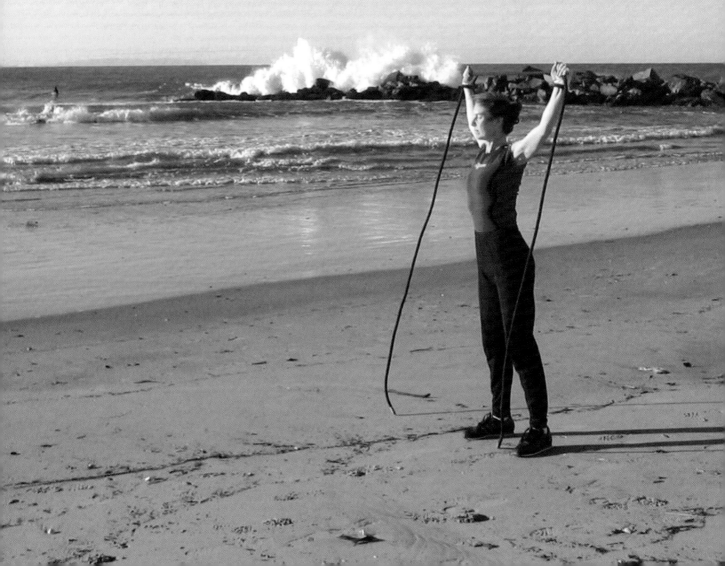

Unbounded optimism, all flourishing
ਚੜਦੀ ਕਲਾ ਸਰਬਤ ਕਾ ਭਲਾ
Chardi kala, sarbat ka bhala

-Sikh Greeting

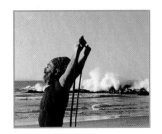

strong
flexible
poised
balanced
aware
optimistic!

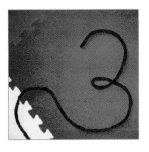

RUSSAYOG SPIRIT

As we travel in our lives, we all face experiences that comfort us, rattle us, or are uninteresting. How we perceive and utilize these experiences differs from person to person. Some people have an unusually comforting string of experiences, while others have very challenging experiences. Nevertheless, the capacity of joy and happiness is almost unrelated to the nature of experiences. Joy and happiness is determined by one's mental and emotional ਭਾਵ (bhav) or attitude. Of course, one needs a certain minimum standard of food, shelter, and love before a human can even think of ਆਨੰਦ (anand) or bliss.

What allows some people to take all challenges in the way a yogi looks at an asan— as a source of growth? The underlying difference is summarized by optimism. An optimistic person focuses on the good that will result from all actions. But what makes a person optimistic? Scientific research shows that some of the optimism has a genetic component. Just as our musculature, mental abilities, etc., has genetic components which we inherit, a part of optimism is inherited. However, just as anyone can improve his/her physique and sharpen his/her mind, life experience and practice can increase the optimism we feel.

Make-Up of the Optimistic View

The central theme of RussaYog is ਚੜਦੀ ਕਲਾ chardi kala (soaring spirit, rising optimism, unbounded optimism). It may be said that RussaYog's business is "nurturing and growing optimism." Every RussaYog session should enhance the practitioner's optimism. Essential to optimism are the mental and physical states described below in the chart. The mind has to feel free, calm, alert, worry-free and capable of resolve. The body has to feel balanced, strong (inside and outside), and flexible.

> RussaYog's business: nurturing and growing optimism.

In the absence of freedom (or at least hope of freedom), in the absence of a strong healthy body (or expectations of one), it becomes difficult to be optimistic. It is also hard to be optimistic if our mind is closed to new ideas.

MIND-BODY FITNESS AND OPTIMISM: TRAINING THE MIND AND BODY

Numerous scientific studies have established that there is a close link between exercise and optimism. While some depressed people have chemical imbalances in their brain which can be helped by prescription drugs, most depressed people can benefit from exercise. Yoga in general and RussaYog in particular adds the calm-alert-mind benefit, making the practice particularly joyful. For a small fraction of the human population the brain appears to be hard-wired from birth in a way that physical activities (play, workouts) provide a sense of pleasure. For most people, however, the connection between fitness and pleasure has to be established. The RussaYog session is particularly suited to develop this fitness-pleasure link. This is because:

- the session is easy to master, so that a novice can do the same session as an expert;
- each student can bring his/her body to its own limit several times during a session, providing a sense of elation and accomplishment; and
- the effects of RussaYog on musculature and overall fitness can be seen within a month of regular practice, providing encouraging feedback.

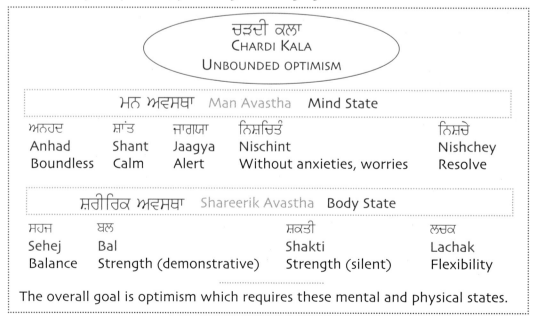

ਚੜਦੀ ਕਲਾ
CHARDI KALA
UNBOUNDED OPTIMISM

ਮਨ ਅਵਸਥਾ Man Avastha   Mind State

ਅਨਹਦ	ਸ਼ਾਂਤ	ਜਾਗਯਾ	ਨਿਸ਼ਚਿੰਤ	ਨਿਸ਼ਚੇ
Anhad	Shant	Jaagya	Nischint	Nishchey
Boundless	Calm	Alert	Without anxieties, worries	Resolve

ਸ਼ਰੀਰਿਕ ਅਵਸਥਾ Shareerik Avastha   Body State

ਸਹਜ	ਬਲ		ਸ਼ਕਤੀ	ਲਚਕ
Sehej	Bal		Shakti	Lachak
Balance	Strength (demonstrative)		Strength (silent)	Flexibility

The overall goal is optimism which requires these mental and physical states.

RussaYog: A Tool

The RussaYog experience is a simulation of relaxing, joyful, and stressful conditions using ropes and yogic principles. The experience is designed to prepare you for real life experiences arising in family life, relationships at work and at home. The goal is to help you face predictable and unpredictable situations with calmness and optimism. If a situation is predictable, a yogic mind should be able to see it coming and prepare for it. If the situation is unpredictable, yogic mind refrains from self-pity and blame and tries to make the best of it. Thus the RussaYog session is not an end to itself—it is a tool to face life's challenges and build pathways for growth. The use of mudra, asan, vishram, as described later, allows one to train oneself for life's opportunities.

RUSSAYOG: NOT JUST A FITNESS PROGRAM

RussaYog develops an extremely strong, a flexible, and balanced body. However, what really distinguishes it is the mind-body balance it creates. This is very important, since so many fitness programs can result in injuries and subsequent long term health problems. In most fitness programs that involve competitive sports injury through contact or overuse is nearly guaranteed. To avoid injury one has to essentially discontinue the sport. Consider the following:

Running: A great activity for stress relief and heart-lung fitness, but will usually result in injuries related to knees, hips,ankles, and back.
Basketball: A good, fun sport which develops excellent hand-eye coordination and physical fitness. Common injuries are related to knees and ankles.
Volleyball: A great workout for leg strength and quickness. However, if you have regularly spiked the ball, then you can understand why the shoulders pay the price.
Tennis: Good fitness exercise. Wrists, elbows, and shoulders are vulnerable.
Skiing: A thrilling experience, good for strength and stamina. If you are lucky only the knees will suffer. If you are unlucky, a fall or collision can hurt everywhere.
Golf: Get fresh air, bond with buddies, and develop strategy. Back, shoulders, and wrists pay the price.
Cycling: A great stamina builder. Shoulder pain, hip and knee issues can be serious. For men, too much cycling can lead to fertility issues as well.
Swimming: A wonderful exercise to build strength and stamina. Shoulders can be troubled, especially if you swim competitively.
Soccer: A great team sport that is exciting and builds speed and stamina. Knees and hips pay the price, unless there are collisions. The injuries from contact sports like rugby and football are well known. Consider 50-year old man who has played football or rugby competitively; note the impact of these sports on the human body.

Clearly if one is to avoid injury, one has to 1) be aware of one's body signals and take action; 2) be wise to end one sport and pick up a different sport. In the United States 120,000 hip replacements and 245,000 knee replacement surgeries are performed each year. Of course not all of these are sports related—most are due to obesity-related issues. But even top rated athletes are now requiring these surgeries before they turn 50. It is expected that nearly 6% of U.S. population will eventually need knee replacements and 3% will need hip replacements.

A key part of the RussaYog session is the preparation including pranayam (breathwork) where the mind is activated to be in a calm-alert state so the possibility of injury is minimized. The use of ropes to hold onto also makes injuries less likely. One uses the rope as a partner, entering the pose with deliberation and confidence.

> A key part of the RussaYog session is the preparation... where the mind is activated to be in a calm-alert state so the possibility of injury is minimized.

CALM-ALERT AND CALM-RELAXED STATE

An important goal of yoga mind/body fitness is to learn how to bring the mind to a high level of alertness while staying calm and, at will, bringing the mind to a relaxed state. The calm-alert state is needed when one is under stress. The calm-alert state channels the body's energies to more efficiently deal with stress. Panic, anxiety, fear, and hopelessness are negative reactions to stress and are avoided in the calm-alert state. It is equally important to learn to be in the calm-relaxed state when there is no stress. Often one dissipates energy through worry, unnecessarily wasting mental and physical resources.

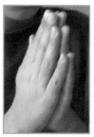

YOG ਜੋਗ: Coherent Union

Yog or union, or more precisely, coherent union, and yogabhyas or practice of yoga is fast becoming an important tool for coping with the stresses of life. Its purpose goes beyond just stress relief. It allows you to accomplish goals with minimal effort using the principles of coherent action. When we talk of coherent union what do we mean? Union of what? On a physical level the union is between our muscles, lungs, heart, bones, tendons, etc., so we have a balanced, harmonious body. On a mental level our thoughts are imaginative, yet in coherence with reality. And our thoughts and physical actions are in coherence. On a social and spiritual level where we see ourselves as part of greater humanity and the Universe.

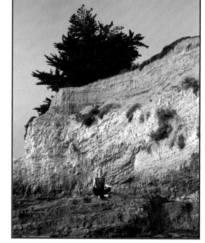

The benefit of such a coherent union results in less negative stress in our lives. We reach a state where our body is truly healthy and we minimize the cycle of health-sickness-medicine, health-sickness-medicine, remaining more in tune with our body's needs. We reach a state where worry and fear do not dominate our mind, and where "me-versus-you" battles do not eat up our precious life.

RussaYog Philosophy

The mool mantra (core concept) of Sri Guru Granth Sahib is the inspiration for RussaYog.

IkOnkar: One source, many manifestations. All life is interconnected. My happiness is not based on your misery. Your wellness improves my health.

SatNam: By understanding and incorporating universal truth—scientific, social, spiritual (of which love for all is the central one)—I can reach a state of harmony.

Nirvair: By eliminating the negativity of prejudice, hatred, fear, and anger I balance my mind and body.

Gur Parsad: I seek Truth from the Universe; eyes and mind open and alert.

ਚੜਦੀ ਕਲਾ

Arrogance, anxiety, and despair replaced by chardi kala (unbounded optimism).

Harnessing Gravity

Prakriti (Nature) has ensured that growth occurs when we go outside our comfort zone—under stress. For proper growth the response to stress should be positive. Several systems of yoga have been developed with specific emphasis on physical discipline, mental discipline, and spiritual discipline. The general principle of yogic postures (or asans) is quite simple—place your body in a difficult motionless state and then use breathwork and mind control to maintain calmness.

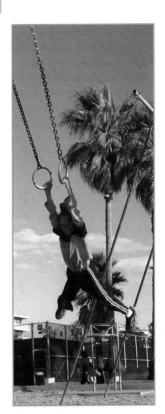

Accessories or props are rarely used for yoga, and then only to assist in making some asans more achievable (or more difficult). This adds to the simple beauty of yoga (just your body and Earth—in balance). To reach the state of crisis, or to go beyond your comfort zone, the traditional yoga asans have to become increasingly difficult. Complicated body positions, like twists, are added, or risky inversion positions are performed. If the body is not well prepared, it is possible to become injured in these asans. The use of a russa (rope) allows the yogi to step outside the comfort zone in just three or four breaths with minimal risk of injury.

Over the past four decades I have developed and used RussaYog or Rope-Yoga. RussaYog is designed to bring the user to the four mind states described above. By adding a rope thrown over an anchor the yogi can practice powerful asans where it is possible to reach the "crisis level" (i.e., you may find your body trembling) in just a few breaths. The free flowing rope, held in each hand, coupled with powerful yogic asans allows us to use gravity to create stresses that are

23

not possible by traditional asans. It is thus possible to reach one's own limits in balance, flexibility, and strength rapidly, yet safely. As in traditional yoga, one then uses breathwork and a heightened mind-awareness to retain calm in this state.

ਰਸਾਂ RUSSA (ROPE)

A word about the russa, or rope. Any rope will do for RussaYog, but some are preferable, depending upon the size of a person's hand, and his/her comfort with gripping. The rope shown in the photos is made of jute. It is quite flexible and feels natural. One can use weight-lifting gloves during the workout until the grip strength builds up and the bare rope feels fine. A one-inch thickness seems perfect for many people and because of it's natural fiber, jute provides a good grip without having to wrap the rope.

> By adding a rope...
> the yogi can practice
> powerful asans where
> it is possible to reach
> the "crisis level"
> in just a few breaths.

The rope is free-flowing and anchored over a sturdy length of round wood, or a branch, or a beam which is securely anchored and can hold the student's body weight. On a Primal Shakti Yoga Tree the rope is looped around the top bar.

As the Russa-Yogi will immediately sense, the asans will demand strength and balance that will challenge the mind and body. The asans can offer challenges to a person who has just enough strength to stand up from a lying position by holding onto ropes. Yet the asans can also offer challenges to the strongest Olympic athlete as well. In fact the asans are designed to allow one to exercise muscles at a level that even exercise machines, costing thousands of dollars, cannot.

Russayog Primal Shakti: Building Blocks

Four versions of the RussaYog Prima Shakti® Workouts have been designed to suit different needs. All have the same underlying theme, but emphasize different components of the four building blocks, representing life's four stages:

   1) Garabh-lila, birth dance/drama, uses breathwork to calm the mind;
   2) Bal-lila, child's play, develops a powerful, flexible, balanced body;
   3) Veer-lila, warrior dance/drama, based on powerful asans or postures; &
   4) Nirvan, merger dance/drama, where recovery takes place.

The yogi must strive for the reflective mind. While viewing a life situation unfolding a reflective mind can see how the past has led to this event in the now and how his or her response will impact the future. Compare this to a Grandmaster of chess who can see the present setting of chess pieces and read the past, and determine how any move will impact the evolution of the game. A reactive mind reacts to the same event with disregard to past or future and invariably makes a wrong choice.

A reflective mind is particularly critical in stressful situations whereby the response is calm, not based on anger or panic or frustration. A reflective mind creates karmas or actions that are graceful and harmonious. Once you have trained your mind to be reflective it does so effortlessly, like a child riding a swing. A trained child almost effortlessly pumps the swing at the right moment to get that swing flying.

The veer-lila portion of a RussaYog session takes the yogi and gently places him/her in an asan where gravity is manipulated (through the rope) to create forces in multiple directions. With various forces pulling/pushing in dozens of directions the yogi achieves balance and holds the asan for several deep breaths. The difficulty builds and the mind learns to accept the situation and maintain a coherent balance.

The asans are excellent for building strong posture and core muscles, as well as shoulders, chest, and gripping muscles. At the end of a session the yogi should not only feel a sense of heightened balance and symmetry, but also a "pump" that is usually associated with weight training. The yogi will learn to dissociate from the discomfort and stay in harmony.

In the previous chapter we discussed the four distinct mind-states. The four building blocks of RussaYog are designed to take the yogi through these four mind states.

Lila (Dane-drama)	Man avastha (Mind-state)
Garabh-lila (birth-drama) Bal-lila (the childhood-dance) Veer-lila (the warrior-dance) Nirvana (merger-dance)	Shant (calm) Chanchal (playful) Sthir (focused) Supt (restful)

Primal Shakti® Workouts

There is something primal about ropes that appeals to all of us—from toddlers to teens to adults to the elderly. When children grip ropes they automatically leap and swing and engage in fantasies. When adults grip ropes they can test out their strength and fortitude. For elderly, ropes give an opportunity to be young again. It is joyful to see a person who is limited by Parkinson's illness transform as he grips ropes and does graceful asans, or pull-up squats! Equally joyful is seeing children run to the ropes and leap up.

The RussaYog Primal Shakti workouts with its four dance-dramas can be mixed and matched for all of life's stages. By focusing on bal-lila, along with interspersed asans, teen's young bodies can be strengthened while keeping the workout engaging. By doing the asans gently and, if needed, on a chair, those with limited-mobility can make their bodies stronger, more balanced, and increasingly flexible.

The different versions of Primal Shakti emphasize different combinations of the four stages of RussaYog. The pie charts illustrate an appropriate mixture of the four building blocks. For healthy and fit people (versions I and II); for youth (version III) and for low mobility persons (version IV). Details are described in later chapters.

Garabh-lila (in blue), Bal-lila (Red), Veer-lila (Green), and Nirvan (Yellow)

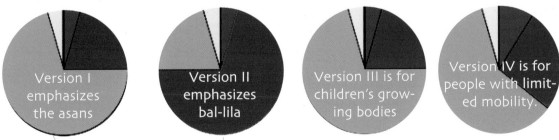

Version I emphasizes the asans — Chapters 4,5,6

Version II emphasizes bal-lila — Chapters 4,5,6

Version III is for children's growing bodies — Chapter 7

Version IV is for people with limited mobility. — Chapter 8

25

Russayog Primal Shakti® Workouts

Powerful mind-body experiences using a rope, your body, and earth's gravity allow you to develop power, balance, flexibility, and mental calm. The four versions of the Primal Shakti workouts outlined below can be done with fixed anchors across which a rope is looped or with the light and portable Primal Shakti Yoga Tree.

Primal Shakti Version I
Overall mind-body fitness

Focus is on yogis mind-body awareness. Starts with stretches and breathing and a few minutes of power movements. Most of the workout centers around powerful yogic asans done with ropes.

Primal Shakti Version II
For athletes

This workout focuses on power. Develops core strength and balance through rapid, strong movements which involve the entire body. Punctuated by breathwork and a few yogic asans.

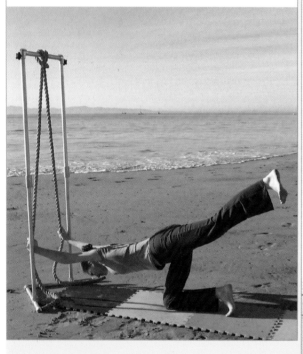

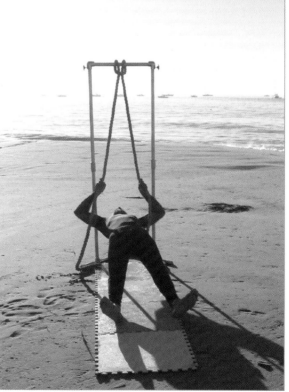

Primal Shakti Version III
For young bodies

Developed specifically for youth. It uses the rope-based exercises to lengthen and strengthen young muscles and improve balance and concentration.

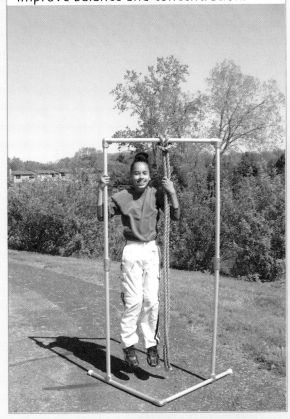

Primal Shakti Version IV
For low-mobility users

Done with the Primal Shakti Yoga Tree, or a fixed anchor, this routine can be done in a chair, if needed.

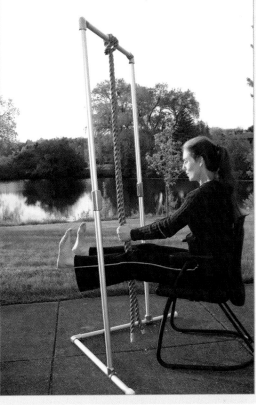

Primal Shakti Yoga Tree® weighs about 15 pounds and fits into a 3 ft. x 10-inch bag.

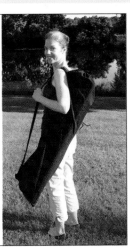

Extended Primal Shakti Yoga Tree® weighs about 20 pounds and fits into a handy carrying bag.

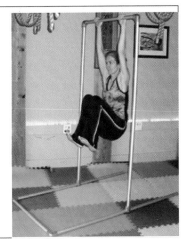

उग्र flexibility धृढ़ strength भाव poise

Dance like no one is watching,
Love like you'll never be hurt,
Sing like no one is listening,
Live like it's heaven on earth.

-William Purkey

No anxiety, Balanced, Optimistic
ਨਿਝਚਿੰਤੰ ਸਹਜ ਚੜਦੀ ਕਲਾ
Nishchint, Sehej, Chardi Kala

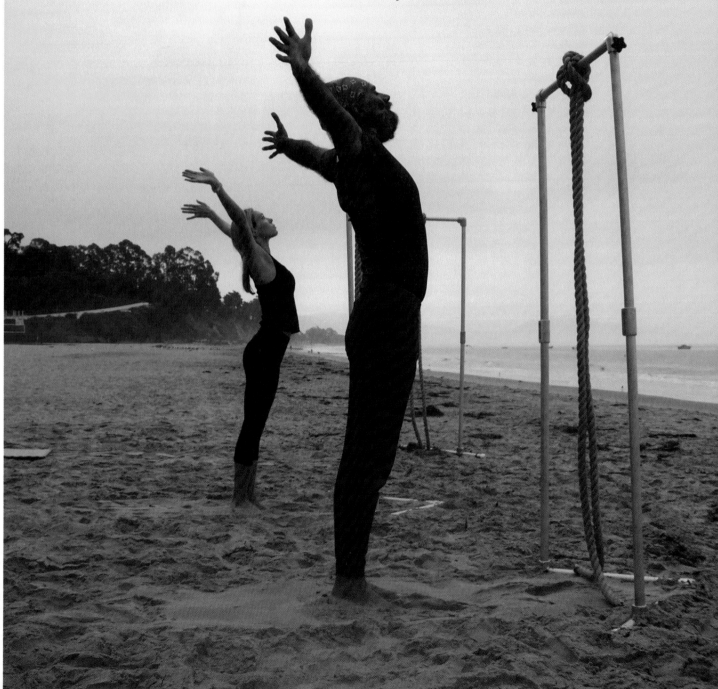

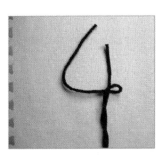

RUSSAYOG:
PREPARATION
AND PRANAYAM

RussaYog: Rituals before Beginning

When you visit a place of worship, you may experience small rituals that have been developed to alter your emotional-mental-physical state. This preparation reminds you that you are about to do something different. Before entering a Sikh Gurdwara (place of worship) you remove your shoes, hand them to a volunteer who greets you and, perhaps, dusts off your shoes. Barefoot, you approach a communal faucet and rinse off your hands and feet. You observe a "message of the day," the first verse that was revealed when the Guru Granth Sahib was opened that morning. You salute others who are gathered there, bowing to the Guru's words. Each small act is a preparation for your mind and body to feel ready for the experience. Rituals are not exclusive to places of worship. If you are an engineer working at an Intel fabrication facility, before entering the clean room, you would perform a series of "rituals." Shoes are removed, booties donned, head is capped, gloves are worn, etc. You mentally review safety and contamination guidelines.

RussaYog is a holistic mind-body experience and should not be undertaken without preparation. Keeping our "eyes on the prize," the yogi wants to emerge in "chardi kala" with a feeling of being energized.

Review these mind-body states. Lighten your mental and physical load. Continually remind yourself of chardi kala until it becomes a constant state of mind.

ਚੜਦੀ ਕਲਾ
chardi kala
unbounded optimism

ਮਨ ਅਵਸਥਾ		Man Avastha	Mind State		
ਅਨਹਦ	ਸ਼ਾਂਤ	ਜਾਗਯਾ	ਨਿਸ਼ਚਿੰਤੰ		ਨਿਸ਼ਚੇ
anhad	shant	jaagya	nischint		Nishchey
boundless	calm	alert	without anxieties/worries		resolve

ਸ਼ਰੀਰਿਕ ਅਵਸਥਾ		Shareerik Avastha	Physical State		
ਸਹਜ	ਬਲ		ਸ਼ਕਤੀ		ਲਚਕ
sehej	bal		shakti		lachak
balance	strength (demonstrative)		strength (silent)		flexibility

---

Loosening Up: Rope Stretches

Before starting a RussaYog session do a few simple stretches which awaken muscles, improve flexibility and strength, and prepare the wrists and forearms for the asans.

THE CLIMB

(BOTH HANDS): Grasp the ropes with both hands straight above your head. Keeping your toes on the ground grasp the rope as high as you can. Feel a deep stretch across your shoulders, upper back, and abdomen. Keeping hold, sway your hip to one side, then another. Hold the stretch for a few breaths.

(ONE HAND): Release the lower hand, letting it hang at your side and feel the stretch along your side. Let your head hang towards the shoulder of your lowered arm. Repeat with the other hand.

YOGA TREE:
Hold top bar as you stretch

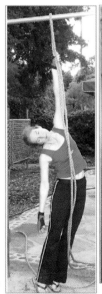

One hand grasps the rope

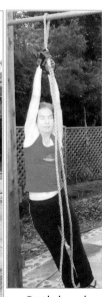

Both hands grasp the rope

LUNGE AND STRETCH: Hold each rope separately with your hands, chest high. Lunge forward with the right leg. Bend your right knee, and bring your arms behind you, gradually straightening your arms, your abdomen reaching forward towards your thigh. Feel a deep stretch across your chest, upper back, and hip. Left calf is also stretched. Hold for 10-15 seconds.

Then do hamstring stretch.

YOGA TREE: DO ALTERNATE STRETCH (BELOW)

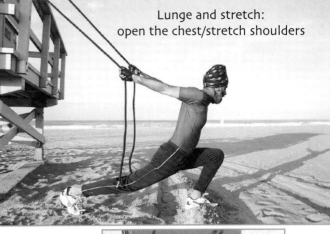

Lunge and stretch:
open the chest/stretch shoulders

HAMSTRING STRETCH: Keeping your feet where they are (see above), slowly raise your upper body and straighten your leg. Keeping your right leg forward, bend your upper body over your straightened right leg. With each exhale, lower your upper body, your abdomen reaching towards your thigh until you feel a deep stretch in the hamstring and hip of the right leg. Use your arms to control the upper body position. No pain should be felt; just a deep stretch. Hold for 10-15 seconds, then slowly raise your upper body and bring your right leg back, next to your left foot.

Repeat with other leg.

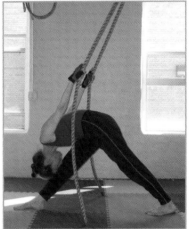

Hamstring stretch

with Primal Shakti Yoga Tree

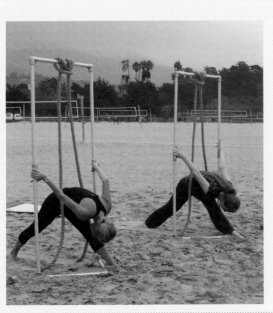

HAMSTRING STRETCH:

HOW TO DO WITH YOGA TREE:

Stand under anchor, hold the Tree on the sides, waist high. Bring one foot forward, on outside of the tree's base. Step back with the other foot a few steps so you have a wide stance. Stretch torso forward with leg straight, holding the Tree with palm facing each other. You may bend elbows. Ease into the stretch by using the sides of the yoga tree to go deeper into the stretch.

FLOOR STRETCH TO STRENGTHEN THE LOWER BACK:

Lie on the stomach, hips directly under the anchor. Hold each rope separately with your hands, about 8-10 inches off the ground. Extend your arms forward, elbows bent,

so the hands are more than shoulder width apart. Pulling down on the rope, lift your upper body. Press the feet together and lift the legs slightly off the ground. Keep the hamstrings and buttocks tense. Keep the head aligned with the spine.
Hold for three deep breaths.

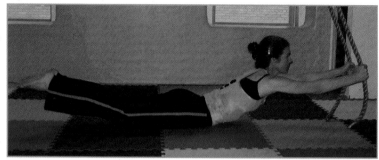

Primal Shakti Yoga Tree

WITH YOGA TREE:
Lie down.
Extend your arms forward to take hold of the rope.
Adjust your position so the ropes fall vertical.
Press down on the ropes, lift the legs, keeping the leg and buttock muscles engaged.
Bend at elbows if there is any shoulder discomfort.

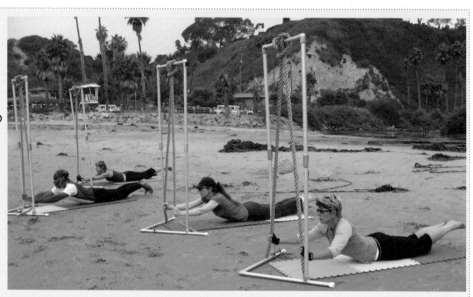

RussaYog Pranayam

Pranayama or breathwork (pran: life; yama: exercise or practice) is an integral part of any yogic session. Pranayama is a powerful tool in our journey to self-awareness and balance. It should be a part of daily routine and will, with practice, become the normal style of breathing. When one observes the breathing style of a healthy child one can see how the child breathes low, ie., presses the belly out and opens the entire chest cavity filling up with air. However, as we get older and are engulfed in an unhealthy atmosphere of loss of trust, fear, panic, anxiety, poor posture, and disease, we start the normal shallow breath we

A key part of the RussaYog session is the preparation, including pranayam, where the mind is activated to be in a clam-alert state so the possibility of injury is minimized.

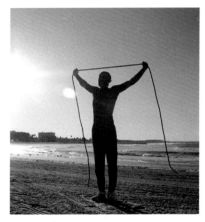

observe in a majority of people. This breath is shallow, using the upper chest movement alone. The pace is rapid (12 breaths a minute or more) and the full capacity of the lungs is not utilized. This doesn't improve even in distance runners or other athletes who may have great stamina. In yoga the breathing is deep and the mind is focused on calmness. In the RussaYog style there are calm breaths as well as breaths with arm movements and stretches. Some of the pranayama sequences are very muscular and allow the yogi to come to a high state of alert and calmness in a minute or two. In all of the pranayama sequences described below (gentle and muscular), the mind is calm and optimistic. We start with breath-work that invokes peace and harmony (shanti) before moving to a different state of alertness in preparation for the yogabhyas (yoga exercises).

Remind oneself, when beginning pranayam, that self-awareness and optimism is the core of the RussaYog session. Maximize the benefits from RussaYog by being in Chardi kala or unbounded optimism. This requires giving up complaints, a sense of victimization, blame, and instead believing that the Universe is constructed in a manner in which we can reach a state of harmony and happiness.

In RussaYog we use a variety of breathing techniques to harness the mind and place it in a very optimistic, joyful, calm, yet alert state. Normally yogic breathing should occur through the nose, but in RussaYog sessions the highly demanding bal-lila and asans require mouth breathing, since one needs a higher oxygen intake. One can slowly learn to get the higher oxygen needed using nose breathing as one becomes more proficient. Mouth breathing should be done in an environment where the air is clean, since the filtering coming from nose breathing is not available when one breathes from the mouth. Apart from the intense parts of RussaYog, nose breathing is utilized during the preparation (mudra) and rest and recovery (vishram) periods.

MENTAL AND EMOTIONAL STATE

Take a few moments to learn to come into the mental and emotional state where you will benefit the most from RussaYog. Many breathing sequences start in Tadasan, so it is useful to review this important pose—Mountain pose.

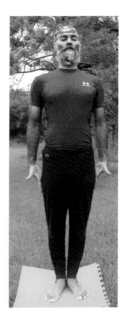

उद्मस्त TADASAN: Stand with feet together, spread your toes and press them into the floor. Pull your kneecaps up to draw strength into your thighs, but do not lock your knees.
Squeeze your buttocks. Pull your shoulders back and down, opening your chest.
Press your hands down and spread your fingers.
Close your eyes, maintaining your balance.
Feel as if your body is light, lifting upward.

BASICS OF THE YOGIC BREATH

ਸ਼ਾਂਤੀ **1. SHANTI (PEACE):** Seated in Sukhasan or standing in a relaxed state, take 5 breaths. Close your eyes and visualize being in harmony.

ਜਾਗ **2. JAAG (AWAKEN):** Visualize yourself awakening to a beautiful moment like a sunrise, springtime, a flower. Stand with hands folded below the abdomen. Raise the arms upwards to the sky inhaling. Reach upwards stretching the body and then exhale bringing the hands down. Repeat for 5 breaths.

ੴ **3. IkOnkar (One source):** This muscular 5-breath sequence ends in a sixth breath in the Namaskar position.
Visualize coming into harmony within yourself and with the Universe.

Breath 1 Visualize harmony within yourself.
Breath 2 Harmony between you and your family/friends.
Breath 3 Harmony in your society;
Breath 4 Harmony in the world;
Breath 5 Harmony in the Universe.

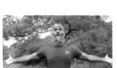

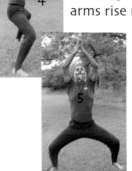

Start in Tadasan. Press your palms into each other just in front of your navel. Take a wide stance and bend at your knees keeping your torso upright.

Breath 1: As you inhale pull your hands down and then upwards reaching and stretching. When your arms are vertical reach up some more. Then slowly bring them down finally ending so your palms are pressed against each other just above your stomach.

Breath 2: Repeat (except the starting position is now higher). Again inhale bringing your arms down and then up. Exhale slowly finally bringing your palms in front of your chest.

Breath 3: Repeat except you are now starting with your palms higher. Breath 3 ends with your palms pressed just above your shoulder height.

Breath 4: Repeat and end the breath with your palms pressed just above your head.

Breath 5: Inhale as you open your arms. As your arms rise up, straighten your legs. Finish the fifth breath with your palms pressed in the Namaskar position in front of your chest. Press your palms in, standing strong, chest lifted. Inhale. Exhale bringing your arms down, stretching.

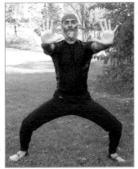
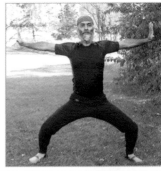

ਸ਼ਕਤੀ 4. SHAKTI (INNER STRENGTH)
Begin by visualizing power flowing in your body. Every cell in your body is infused with power and strength.
Stand in Tadasan. Extend your arms forward. Pull your palms up and spread the fingers. Take a wide stance, bend the knees, and keep your back vertical. While inhaling, pull your (straightened) arms to the sides, opening your chest. Briefly hold and bring your arms back while exhaling. Repeat three times.

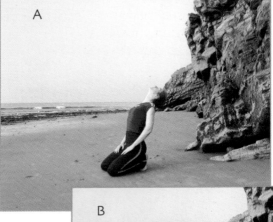

A

ਨਿਸ਼ਚੇ 5. NISHCHEY (RESOLVE)
Train your mind to make a commitment and not abandon your commitments.
This pranayam is useful for restoring elasticity to the abdominal muscles, and enhancing digestive efficiency.
Kneel and sit on your heels.
If comfortable, turn your toes facing forward stretching the bottom of your foot,or place a rolled up blanket under the thighs, or sit on a chair and place the palms on the thighs.
The palms of the hands are resting on the thighs.
Fold forward in preparation.
Open your body leaning backward as you inhale (A).
Fold forward as you exhale.
Without inhaling suck in your stomach pressing it inward and hold for about 8 seconds (B). Repeat for 2-3 breaths.

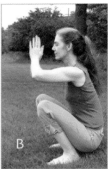

B

ਸਹਜ 6. SEHEJ (BALANCE)
In this pranayam visualize your mind and body poised and balanced.
No negative emotions exist within.
You are highly aware of every muscle in your body.
Sit on your feet with heels on the ground.
Place your arms on your knees, pull your palms up, raise your chest and prepare (A).
Raise your palms up in Namaskar position (B).
Squeeze in and take one breath.

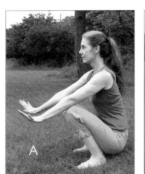

A   B

If you are short on time or want to do 2-minutes of pranayam during your workday you can pick the sequences that suit you. Once you are done with pranayam, stand in tadasan and again focus on the mind-body states described in the table at the start of this chapter.

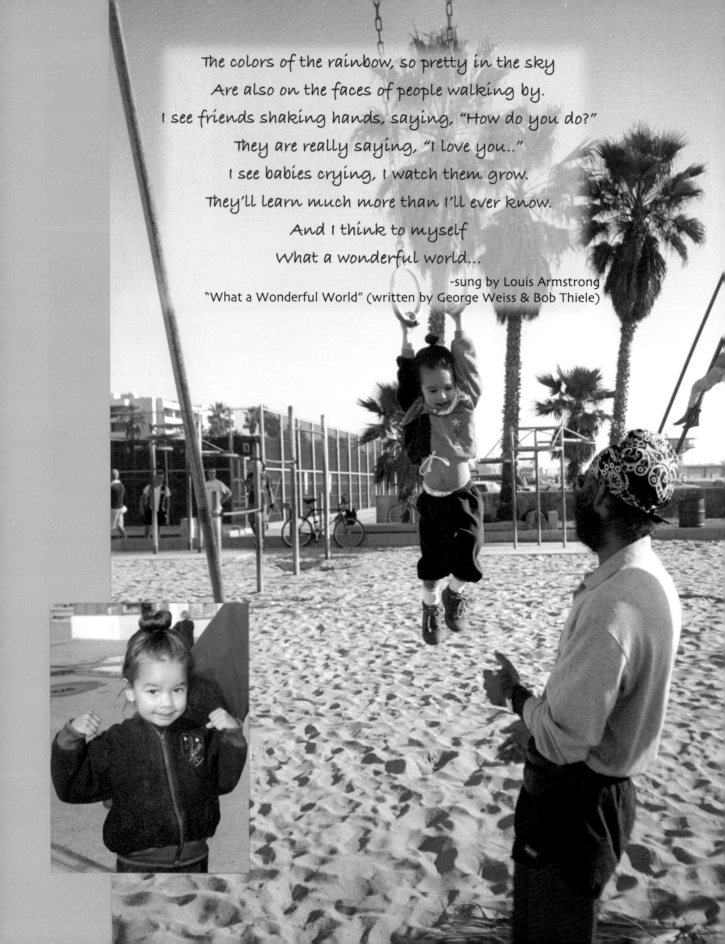

The colors of the rainbow, so pretty in the sky
Are also on the faces of people walking by.
I see friends shaking hands, saying, "How do you do?"
They are really saying, "I love you.."
I see babies crying, I watch them grow.
They'll learn much more than I'll ever know.
And I think to myself
What a wonderful world...

-sung by Louis Armstrong
"What a Wonderful World" (written by George Weiss & Bob Thiele)

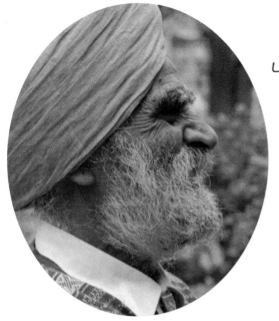

Lowering your threshold for pleasure!

The King of Bal-lila: Laughter!

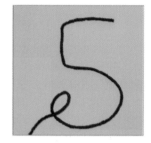

RUSSAYOG: BAL-LILA

The RussaYog yatra (journey) now moves onto Bal-lila (childhood's dance/drama). The man-avastha (mind state) is chanchal and full of joy and anticipation. The workout is done with and without ropes and, depending upon the needs, could be for 8-10 minutes or up to 30-40 minutes. Bal-lila is essential to develop strong, long muscles, flexibility, and balance. As noted in Chapter 3, the proportion of Bal-lila can vary, depending upon the abilities/desires of the yogi.

Bal-lila with Ropes and Fixed Anchor

If the ropes are on a fixed stable anchor the yogi doesn't have to pay much attention to body movements forward or sideways. There is a greater ability to do a wider variety of movements.

Bal-lila with Ropes on Primal Shakti Yoga Tree

With a yoga tree the ropes need to be always in the area formed by the side bars (a few degrees off this plane is fine). This causes the yogi to be more focused on the initial body and shoulder positioning so the yoga tree remains stable. The presence of the side bars, however, provide unique and powerful exercise sequences, since the ropes can be wrapped outside the bars and then held.

BAL-LILA
(Man Avastha: Chanchal)

This part of the session uses large, playful movements in order to warm up the muscles and joints, preparing for the next stage. By using the rope the entire body can work harmoniously without stressing your joints. Bal-lila starts with the following sets of exercises. The user can chose exercises depending upon needs and abilities.

NEVER do movements that cause pain.

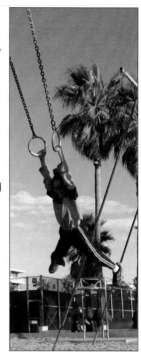

1) Sideways Butterfly Lunge-Stretch

(leg strength, balance, arm strength, hip flexibility)

1: Stand in a wide side stance looking forward, left foot pointing to your left, right foot pointing forward. Stretch arms wide and inhale.
2: While exhaling and twisting towards the left, bend at the left knee keeping the torso upright, bringing the hands forward.
Press your hands together, keeping the right leg straight.
3: Inhale while extending your straight arms back, stretching and opening up your chest, keeping your lower body in the fixed position.
4: exhale bringing your arms back in front of you, pressing your hands in.
The lower body does not move.
5: Inhale, pressing your hips back to the beginning position, stretching your arms, looking forward.
Repeat 10 times.
Then repeat on the other side (right leg bending).

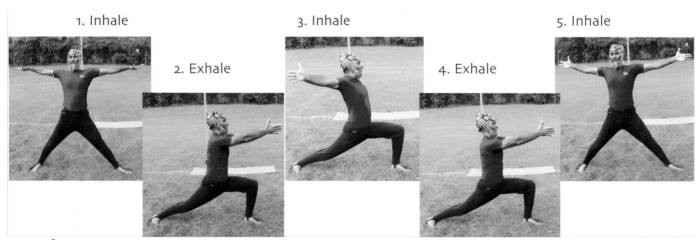

1. Inhale 2. Exhale 3. Inhale 4. Exhale 5. Inhale

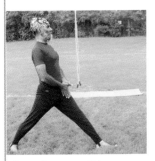

Starting position

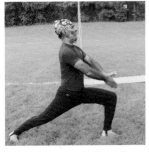

Lunge, press hands

2) Forward Lunge Stretches

(lower body strength, balance, arm strength, flexibility)

Begin with a wide stance, left foot in front pointing forward, right foot behind you pointing to the right. Bend at your left knee, keeping the right leg straight and torso upright. Do not let left knee go beyond the toes.

Press your hands in tight just above the knee.

While inhaling, reach back, straightening the left leg, opening your arms, stretching your shoulders and chest.

Exhale bending your left knee, bringing your hands forward a little higher than the starting position.

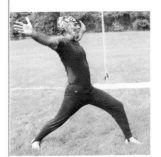

Open arms

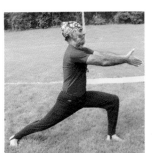

Lunge, hands higher

Repeat, each time bringing your hands up a little higher until your hands are almost vertical.

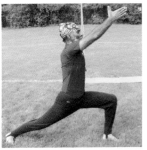

Open arms

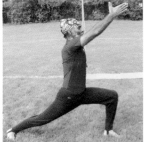

Lunge, hands higher

Then continue bringing your hands downward with each lunge.

Do about 10 lunges on the left knee and 10 lunges on the right knee.

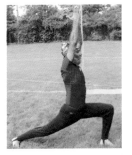

Open arms

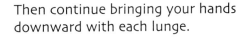

Hands above head

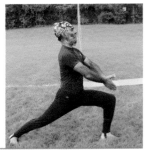

End position

3) Pull-ups/half-squats

(biceps, shoulder, thighs, quickness):

Stand with feet shoulder-width apart, just behind the rope. Hold ropes head level. (A) Keep chest lifted, squat. (B) Use arms and thighs to raise the body. Squeeze the buttocks as you stand, shoulders not hunched.
Do 15 to 30 times.

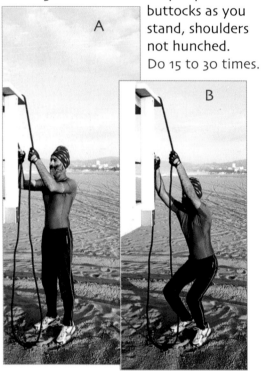

4) Press-down/half-squats

(triceps, shoulder, thighs, quickness):

Hold the rope so both hands are at navel level (C).
Squat down (D) then, using the legs and the pressing (downward) action of the arms, stand up.
Do 15-30 squats.

Pull-ups/half-squats
Use same technique as above.

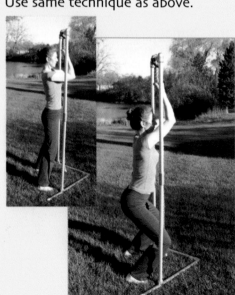

Press-down/half-squats
Lean forward slightly. Squeeze the buttocks, keep shoulders relaxed.

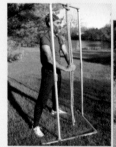

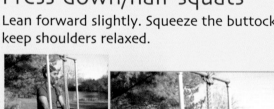

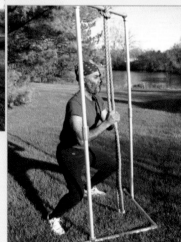

Repeat 30 squats each.

5) Kick Back

(hamstrings, shaping buttocks):

The arms, thighs, and buttocks will be somewhat tired by now, so the next set of exercises uses a different set of muscles.

Before moving to the next set do some kick-backs.

Kick back so the heel hits the buttock.

Alternate for about 30 seconds.

This is a good fatigue-remover and develops a spring to your step.

6) Front Lunge

(chest, arms, thighs, flexibility):

With feet below the anchor, hold the ropes at chest level.

Open the arms to the sides and then lunge forward in a controlled manner.

Squeeze the forearms together as you return to the standing position.

Alternate with each leg for 10-20 lunges.

(ONLY WITH FIXED ANCHOR)

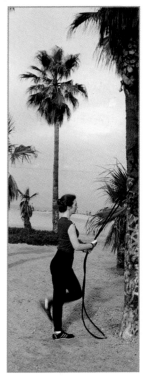

Kick back

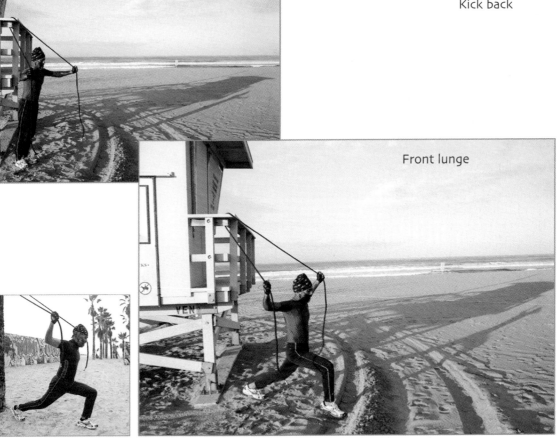

Front lunge

7) High Front Sweeps

(upper thighs, hamstrings, knees, abdominal muscles):
Firmly plant yourself on the left foot.
Place the right foot about 12-18 inches behind the left one.
Tighten the buttocks and thighs and,
holding the ropes for balance in each hand,
sweep the right leg out in a forward motion.

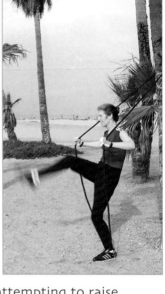

with Primal Shakti Yoga Tree

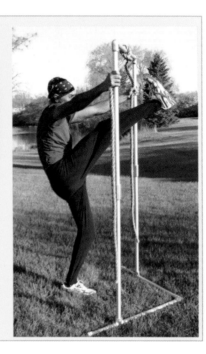

Hold onto the
bars of the
tree while
sweeping the
leg forward.

Do 5-15 sweeps, attempting to raise
the leg higher each time.
Repeat with the other leg 5-15 times.

8) Side Lunges

(ONLY WITH FIXED ANCHOR)

(upper back, biceps, thighs, shoulders):
Stand under the anchor.
Hold the rope at chin level with hands together,
left hand on top. Using hands and keeping the
left foot fixed do a side lunge. Use arms, lats
(upper back), legs, and thighs to come back to a
standing position. Tighten the buttocks as you
stand. Repeat 5-15 times.

Repeat with the other leg 5-15 times.

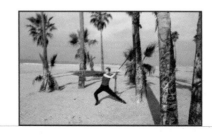

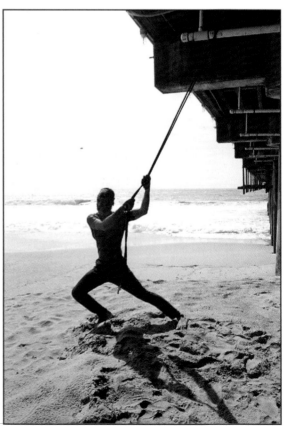

9) Side Leg Raises

(outer thighs, flexibility):
Stand under the anchor.
Hold the ropes for balance.
Raise one leg out to the side, bending the body.
Keep buttock tight.
>   Do 10-15 leg raises.
>   Repeat with the other leg.

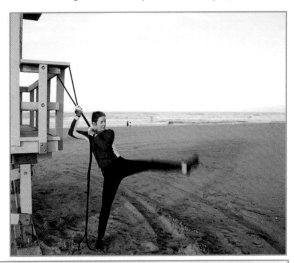

9) WITH THE YOGA TREE

Hold the top bar,
or the sides of the tree.
Raise one leg out to the side,
bending the body.
>   Do 10-15 leg raises.
>   Repeat with the other leg.

10) Back Extension

(lower back, shoulders, buttocks):
Lie on the stomach under the anchor. Take both ropes
in the right hand, 6-12 inches off the floor. Pull down
on the rope, raising the chest and lift the opposite leg.
Exhale as you raise the leg.
>   Do 10 repetitions.
>   Repeat on the other side.
May do with both hands forward holding the ropes, raising both legs.

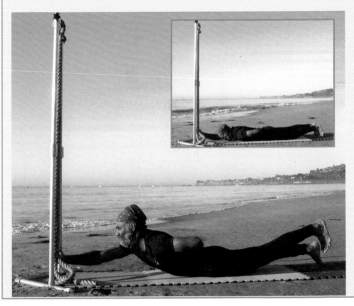

WITH THE YOGA TREE
Lie on the stomach behind the rope
so that the hand with outstretched
arm is able to grip the rope as the
rope falls vertically.
Do not pull the rope towards
you; keep it vertical!
Pull down on the rope, lifting the
chest, exhaling & raising the
opposite leg.
>   10 repetitions each side.

with Primal Shakti Yoga Tree

11) Standing Knee Lifts

(core, upper back, triceps, shoulders):
Stand with one foot under the anchor. Other foot back 1-2 feet, foot pointed at an angle. Hold each rope waist high. Bend front knee, leaning the body towards the rope. Keep pressing down on the rope, strengthening the chest, arms, abs. Raise the forward knee to the hands, exhaling.

Do 10-15 leg raises. Repeat with the other leg.

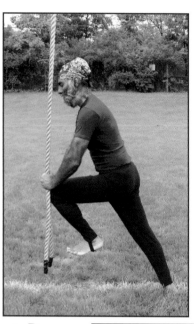

WITH THE YOGA TREE
Same as fixed anchor.

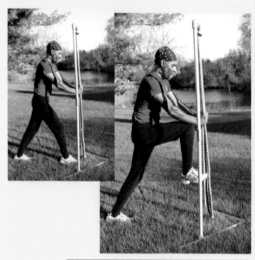

Ropes wrapped around the bar.

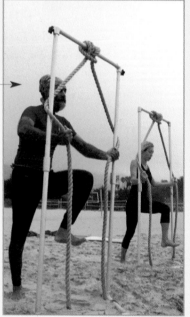

with Primal Shakti Yoga Tree

12) Jump-Float Down

(thighs, upper back, biceps, shoulders):
Feel like a kid again!
Take the ropes at the forehead.
Squat down and lift yourself off the ground.
Float back down gently, with control.

Repeat 10 times.

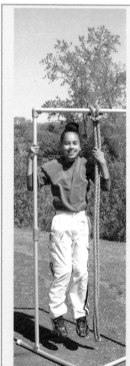

See Chapter 7:
RussaYog Youth Sequence

WITH YOGA TREE
Hold the rope with one hand and the bar with the other. Or, if you are tall enough, hold the top bar with both hands. Squat down, jump up, float back down.
10 times.

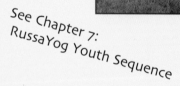

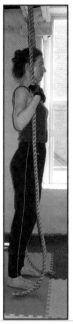

13) Giant Pendulum Swing (Tricep extension/Pull-up)

Stand under the rope, with the feet 6-10 inches apart.

Wrap each side of the rope in each hand at the shoulder level.

Tighten the buttocks and fall forward in a controlled manner keeping the feet fixed.

Elbows are bent, close to the head.

Pull back to standing position and then lean your body back, keeping the body straight, and straighten the arms.

Pull up to a standing position.

   Repeat 5-10 times.

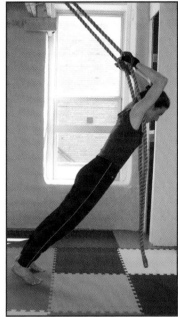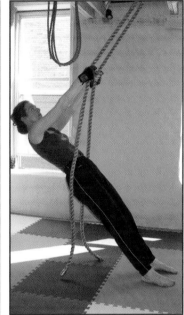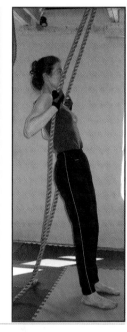

14) Pull-ups from Knees

(Biceps, core):

Kneel under the anchor,
feet separated and toes curled under.

Hold the ropes just above your head.

Keeping the buttocks tight, abdominal muscles engaged, pull yourself up so the upper arms are almost horizontal.

Exhale as you pull up, inhale as you lower yourself.

   Repeat 5-10 times.

SAME WITH YOGA TREE AND FIXED ANCHOR.

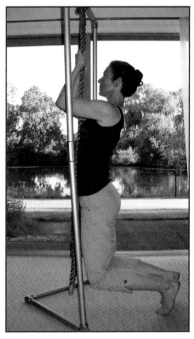

45

15) Pull-up from Floor

(Biceps, core):
Lie under the anchor, feet shoulder-width apart or more, flat on the floor. Reach up and hold the ropes high. Keeping the thighs and buttocks tight, pull yourself up so the elbows face out, chest lifted. Exhale as you pull up, inhale as you lower yourself.
   Repeat 5-10 times.

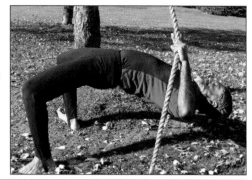

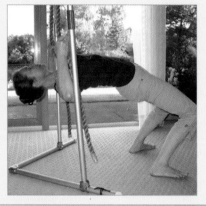

with Yoga Tree

15a) Pull-up from Floor

(Biceps, core):
Lie under the anchor so your shoulders are even with the sides of the tree, feet shoulder-width apart or more, flat on the floor. Reach up and hold the ropes high. Keeping the thighs and buttocks tight, pull yourself up so the elbows face out along the sides of the tree, chest lifted. Exhale as you pull up, inhale as you lower yourself.
   Repeat 5-10 times.

16) Push-ups

(Arms, chest, shoulders):
Lie on the stomach, extending the legs, feet a few inches apart. Palms on the floor, fingers facing forward, elbows bent. Curl toes under. Strengthen buttocks, thighs, arms, back. Press hands into the floor as you lift the body, keeping it straight.
   Repeat 10-12 push-ups.

Modification: you may do push-ups from the knees.

17) Sit-Stand-Sit

(Overall strengthening and balance):
Sit beneath the anchor, feet on the floor, a bit apart.
Hold each rope in each hand, over the head.
Pull yourself up to a standing position.
Then lower yourself to a sitting position.
Try to make the motion smooth, without much wobbling to and fro.
   Repeat 10-12 times.

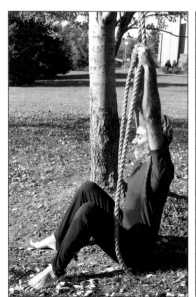

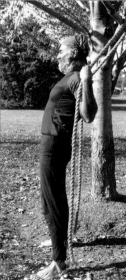

18) Leg Raises from Floor

(Arms, core):
Sit behind the rope so the ropes fall at your knees. Hold the ropes mid-torso height, arms straight. Pull down on the ropes, crunching the abs. Flex the feet, squeeze the buttocks. Without leaning back, lift the legs, exhaling. Release and inhale.
   Repeat 10-20 times.

WITH YOGA TREE: keep ropes vertical.

Modification: you may bend the knees as you lift the legs.

Legs separated

Legs & feet together

with Primal Shakti Yoga Tree

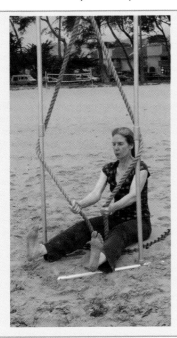

18a) Alternate Leg Raises from Floor

(Arms, chest, core):
Use the same positioning as the leg raises, and instead wrap each rope around the side of each bar.
Take each rope in each hand, pulling your hands toward each other, but not touching the hands to each other.
Pull down on the ropes, crunching the abs.
Flex the feet, squeeze the buttocks.
Without leaning back, lift the legs, exhaling.
Release and inhale.
   Repeat 10-20 times.

Modification: To reduce strain on the lower back, you may bend the knees as you lift the legs. And/or sit on a blanket to elevate the hips

In the playful Bal-lila where the mind is in the chanchal (playful, sampling) state, the yogi will bring the heart rate and breathing efficiency to a level of a mountain climber. And like a mountaineer the yogi will not only use the big hip and thigh muscles, but use pulling muscles (biceps, forearms), pushing muscles (triceps, shoulders, lats), squeezing muscles (chest, side and front abdominals). In a matter of less than ten minutes the yogi will have worked as though having climbed the equivalent of a 20 story building.

At the end of Bal-lila the muscles are engorged with blood, the joints have been warmed up, and ligaments are more flexible. Bal-lila is the winter storm on the Pacific Northwest. The waves have crashed and the surf has dazzled. Now it is time for focus and balance.

Bal-lila...the waves have crashed and the surf has dazzled.

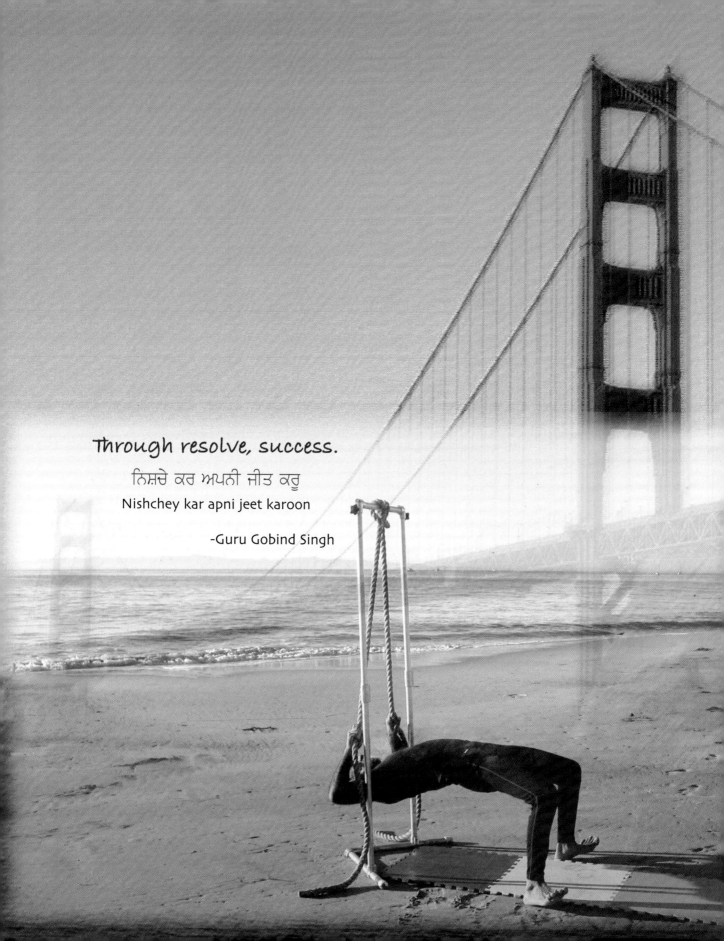

Through resolve, success.

ਨਿਸ਼ਚੇ ਕਰ ਅਪਨੀ ਜੀਤ ਕਰੂੰ

Nishchey kar apni jeet karoon

-Guru Gobind Singh

Imagine the perfect vacation.

Your mind is filled with anticipation. You discover new sensations.

You challenge yourself mentally and physically.

You resolve to seek new sources of joy.

You discover the power of relaxation. You return energized.

This is the RussaYog getaway —enjoy the trip!

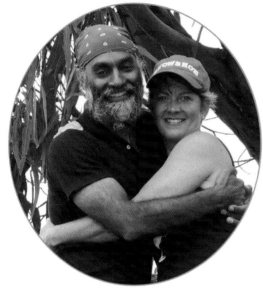

The King of all Asans: The Hug!

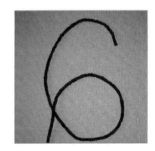

RUSSAYOG: VEER-LILA

INTRODUCTION

The yogi's dance-drama has now moved into the warrior phase. But this is not the wild, uncontrolled warrior. For this warrior time holds still so every muscle, every breath, every neural twitch can be calmly observed and total balance achieved. Veer is the participant and the observer. The yogi senses the pull of mother Earth challenging the muscles. You observe the tension running from the fingers to the forearms to the shoulders to the abdomen to the groin to the thighs to the calf on down to the Earth. The feeling starts from "this is not so bad" to "my muscles are getting a great workout" to "I can't bear the ache any longer" to "I am going to crash right now!" Yet, with practice the yogi learns to use Earth's pull to create balance and harmony—and yes—a beautiful body.

In the beginning, the yogi's mind is barely able to keep the body from collapsing.

However, in a few lessons the mind does start reaching the detached-attached state. The participant and observer mode. Can the yogi take this state of sehej (complete balance) outside the ashram (the yoga studio) into the "real world" of offices, deadlines, children, shopping...? Therein will lie the success of the abhyas (exercise).

Veer-lila corresponds to the adult phase of our lives. A phase where we make commitments—and keep them. We take on challenges and fulfill them—or at least try our best. We grow ourselves as multi-dimensional human beings. We have a strong core, flexibility, strength, and stamina.

The asans of the veer-lila (both with ropes and without ropes) are chosen to place the mind-body in chardi kala—unbounded optimism. As noted in Chapter 3, this requires both emotional and physical well being.

Veer-lila involves stepping outside one's comfort zone in order to grow. During veer-lila the goal of the yogi is to reach the state of dhyan, or meditative awareness. This is the sthir avastha, the coherent state, where distracting diffuse thoughts are channeled to produce a highly focused mind. The performance of each asan involves three part. These are:

i) the veer mudra, in which you energize your body before starting the asan. Begin an asan only when you are prepared physically and emotionally;

ii) the yog-asan which places the body in a state where you are taken outside your comfort zone. Pranayama, or breathwork, allows you to face the asan with confidence and vigor, and drishti, or sight, allows you to focus; and

iv) vishram, rest, allows you to recover and focus for the next asan. Vishram could involve stretches.

PREPARATION FOR THE ASANS
We will review some of the important techniques that should be used to carry out the veer-lila asans in a strong and graceful manner.

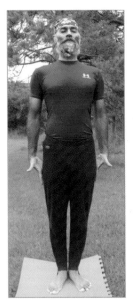

VEER MUDRA
In many asans it is important to begin in the Veer Mudra, or Warrior State. This implies a strong state of commitment. Before starting each asan mentally survey the sequence you are about to follow, start with a strong posture, focus on what is to be done, and take a couple of deep breaths. Energize your body. Feel like the rope is a part of your body. Feel powerful and energized. Maintain not just a physical focus, but also a mental focus before, during, and after each asan—until the entire session is over. RussaYog is not a competitive sport—you need not try to "best" the person next to you. Use your mental focus to do the best asan you can.

USE OF THE MUSCLES DURING AN ASAN
The asans in a RussaYog session are quite demanding if done at the

higher difficulty level. The muscles used during an asan can be divided into two types:
1. active supportive and
2. silent supportive.

The active supportive are muscles that are absolutely needed to maintain the asan—otherwise you will lose your balance and crash. Typical active supportive muscles would be the wrist and forearm muscles for gripping, the thigh and calf muscles for balancing the body, the shoulder and biceps for pulling, etc. Each asan is designed to place stress on the muscular and skeletal structure through active-supportive muscles.

The silent supportive muscles are also very important and should be exercised during an asan, even though one can perform the asan without them. A common form of using silent supportive muscles is the Kegel exercise, clenching the buttocks. Also lifting the kneecaps upwards, pushing downward into the Earth with the feet, engaging the hands, tucking in the abdominal wall, etc., are critical to a successful asan. The silent supportive asans provide that extra grace in the asan and heighten the mental challenge of the exercise.

> *Each asan is designed to place stress on the muscular and skeletal structure through active-supportive muscles.*

During the asana maintain a deep breathing rhythm. If you lose balance or are unable to hold the asan for several breaths, try again. If you find a good balance, close your eyes and mentally "detach" yourself, surveying your posture, as if you are examining yourself from a distance.

A focused concentration is essential for RussaYog. As you prepare for the asan, choose a focal spot to maintain during the entire asan period. It may be a spot on the floor (if you are facing downward), on the wall, or on the ceiling. You may also feel balanced enough to close the eyes during the asan and focus inward.

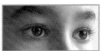

VISHRAM

Once the asan has ended, take a few breaths in a restful state. Rest may mean lying with all the muscles relaxed, or going into child's pose or doing some simple stretches. No thoughts about the asan during the rest. Just relax.

RUSSAYOG'S PLEASURE

Humans are remarkable in that their mental-emotional state can be quite disconnected from the outside world. We can manage to sometimes feel lonely, happy, upset, or joyful, regardless of what is around us. This ability can be exploited to bring yourself to a joyful, optimistic state on demand. That is the goal of RussaYog. So constantly remind yourself of chardi kala and feel the spirits being lifted.

RussaYog strives to take the yogi through a yatra (journey) involving a series of mind-based, emotional and physical experiences so the yogi emerges energized and in chardi kala. The yogi feels light in body and in mind, having worked to discard baggage of worry and anxiety.

Stretching: why does it feel sooo good?
When we look at animals (cats, dogs, panthers...) we see how they recover from fatigue by stretching and holding their stretches for a while. A deep stretch seems to physically rejuvenate us as if someone is squeezing out our fatigue. The emotional benefit of a deep stretch arises from the feeling of pushing to our limits with no one to bind us.

Strong muscles: what makes power feel so good?
Why do we feel good when our muscles are strong and we feel the blood flowing through them (the so-called "pump")? It gives us the sense of being light and unbound. We feel as if nothing is impossible.

Balance: why does it feel so good?
From a four-year old mastering the bicycle to a circus performer, we are all fascinated by balance. After all, life is all about balance. Balance in our body, and also balance at a higher level. Balance between gluttony and starvation; arrogance and subservience; me and you.

VEER-LILA

Preparation—mental, emotional, and physical—is essential for veer-lila asans. Let us remind ourselves of the state we wish to be in—chardi kala—unbounded optimism. The yogi must make sure the mind is free and light. Reflect upon these states:

ਨਿਸ਼ਚਿੰਤ   Nishchint: free of worry

ਨਿਰਵੈਰ   Nirvair: no prejudice

ਸ਼ਾਂਤ   Shant: calm, peaceful

ਜਾਗਿਆ   Jaagya: awake, alert

ਅਨਹਦ   Anhad: no boundaries, free

The body must be strong and ready. Reflect on these physical states:

ਲਚਕ   Lachak: flexibility

ਬਲ   Bal: strength-demonstrative

ਸ਼ਕਤੀ   Shakti: power, silent

ਸਹਜ   Sehej: balance, poise

The RussaYog asans using ropes and some traditional asans are woven together to take the yogi through a ਜਾਤ੍ਰਾ yatra (journey) so one emerges with high spirits.

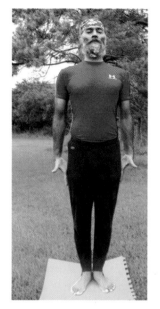

TADASAN

In RussaYog Tadasan (mountain pose) is used continually to rebalance and reset our mind and body.

Press your toes into the floor, strengthen your thighs (but do not lock your knees).

Tighten your buttocks, pull your shoulder back and down.

Press your arms down, spread your fingers and press your hands into your thighs.

Close your eyes.

Feel yourself rising upwards.

Allow all worries and noise from your mind to fade away.

Take 2-3 yogic shant breaths.

RUSSA KICHH (ROPE PULL): PREPARATION

The rope pull is a good way to prepare the mind and body. It allows us to reach deep into our strength and learn to keep our mind calm and alert.

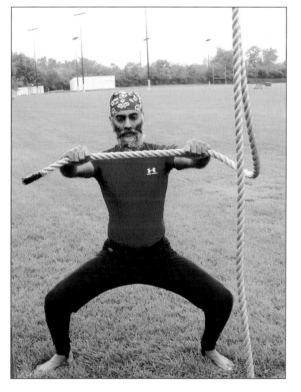

Take one end of the rope with both hands, shoulder-width apart.

Extend your arms forward so they are horizontal.

Take a wide stance and, keeping the torso vertical, bend at your knees.

Pull the rope with each hand using your shoulder strength.

Try to come to your limit (you are almost shaking).

Calm your mind and hold for 2 breaths.

Rise up, take a gentle inhale, keeping your arms horizontal, loosening your grip.

Exhale and release the rope, then stretch by pressing your arms back.

Review the goals of the yogasans and learn about the emotional and physical states of the asans.

Veer-Lila: physical aspects of the asans

Veer-lila asans are designed to create the overall emotional state of chardi kala. They also create a balanced, fit physique. The rope allows us to pull ourselves in various directions, adding strength and balance. In terms of their physical effect, the asans can be categorized thusly:

Physical aspects of the asans				
ਅਨਹਦ	ਸਹਜ	ਆਧਾਰ	ਬਲ	ਵਿਸ਼ਰਾਮ
Anhad Beyond limits Beyond Boundary	Sehej Balance, poise	Aadhar Foundation (core)	Bal Strength	Vishram Restful
Stretching Asans Fosters trust & openness. Lengthens & strengthens muscles.	Improves balance, self-awareness. Helps avoid injuries. Improves body symmetry.	Foundation for core strength (abdominals, lower back, groin, buttocks) Improves posture, sexual and digestive organs. Adds grace & beauty.	Asans to build long, strong muscles of both upper and lower body.	Asans for recovery from fatigue and stress.
Ek, doh, teen Dharat namaskar	Chakar asan	Kaam asan series	Balasan sequence	Child's pose
Ek, doh veer asan	Langar asan	Bridge asan	Abhay	Shoulder stand
Jag namaskar sequence	Teen Dharat namaskar		Agni lapat asans	Hal asan
Trikonasan series	Tadasan		Jhoola asan	Shavasan
Parvat asan			Savaar asan	Pranayam sequences
Inverted stretch				
Garurh Asan				
Seated twist				

Chapter 3 covered the mind-states the RussaYog session takes one into. Our emotions change when we are in the presence of different experiences. A stormy night may create wonder. A healthy baby evokes love. A fellow human in distress induces empathy, etc. The RussaYog asans also involve emotional feelings that should be enjoyed. The ਭਾਵ (bhav) or emotional states that asans place us in are described here:

ਭਾਵ (bhav) EMOTIONAL STATES OF ASANS					
ਖੋਜ Khoj Exploration	ਧਨਵਾਦੀ Dhanwadi Grateful	ਏਕਤਾ Ekta Oneness, harmony	ਵਾਹ Wah Wonder	ਸਹਜ Sehej Balance, poise	ਵਿਸ਼ਵਾਸ Vishvaas Confidence
Build your state of exploring new paths as you reach into directions you normally do not go.	Create a feeling of gratitude as you feel blessed by all that you have and what Earth provides.	Create a sense of harmony throughout the mind and body.	Create a sense of wonder by allowing you to do things that you normally never do. Ropes are perfect for this experience.	Sense of balance and poise is created.	Do something powerful and difficult and imbue yourself with confidence.
Trikonasan series Chakar asans Parvat asan Doh Dharat Namaskar	Ek Dharat namaskar Child's Pose Shavasan	Jag namaskar sequence Inverted stretch Langar asan Bridge asan	Doh, Teen dharat namaskar Abhay Agni lapat Pranayam sequences	Chakar Teen dharat namaskar Jhoola asan	Ek, doh veer asan Kaam asan Agni lapat Balasan sequence Savaar asan

Use every asan to test your limits of strength, balance, and flexibility.
Reflect upon the emotional class of each asan as you perform it.
Depending upon the time available for your practice, choose asans from the list given. Also, it is useful to alternate asans with the rope, and asans without the rope, so your hands can rest from gripping.

You can also punctuate your session with a kriya—a fast-moving exercise with quick breathing.
(see page 99 for an example).

Ek Dharat Namaskar

Emotional class: ਧਨਵਾਦ *dhanwad: gratitude*

Physical class: ਅਨਹਦ *anhad: beyond limit*

Mudra

Fixed anchor
Take the two ropes together in your right hand. Lie down on your stomach with the hips under the anchor. Place your left hand on your lower back (or, if this is uncomfortable, keep it on the floor at your side).

Primal Shakti Yoga Tree
Position yourself so that when you hold the ropes with your right hand extended, the ropes are vertical.

Draw Shakti into your thighs, buttocks, back, chest, arms, and especially triceps. Visualize this asan. Bring your right foot inward and press your toes into the ground.

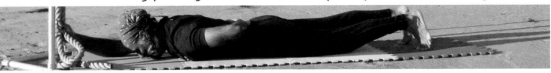

Asan

Pull down on the ropes lifting your chest. Raise your entire left leg off the ground. Stretch, stretch. Feel the strength in your body. Feel the alignment.
Mind is calm, yet alert.
Take 3-4 breaths (35-50 seconds) holding the asan.

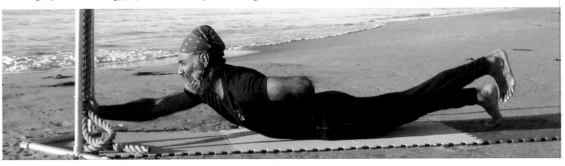

Vishram

Slowly release.
Place your head down, arms in a comfortable position. completely let go of your muscles . Rest for 20 seconds.

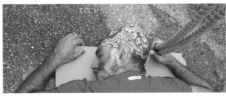

REPEAT ON THE OTHER SIDE (35-50 seconds)

Then come to baalasan—Child's pose—to further relieve the back. Sit back on your heels, tops of feet on the floor, head face down on the floor, arms resting, extended forward on the floor or along your sides with palms facing up. Relax totally.
Feel your emotional/physical stress dissipating.

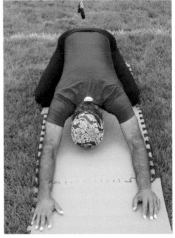

Trikonasan on Knees

Emotional class: ਖੋਜ khoj: explore

Physical class: ਅਨਹਦ anhad: beyond limit

Mudra

Kneel with your knees a little more than shoulder-width apart.
Torso is tall. Toes pointing forward, heels up.
Pull your shoulders back and down.
Draw strength into your body and keep your buttocks tightened.

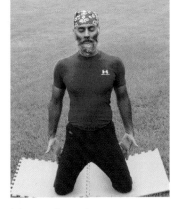

Asan

Slowly start bending to your right. Place your right fingertips on the floor and then slowly raise your left arm up, making a big circle. Extend your left arm towards your right side (don't lean forward or back).

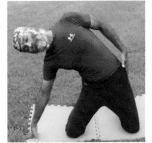 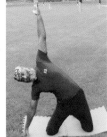

Feel the stretch on your side, and neck.
Hold for 2 breaths.

Return very slowly, reversing your movement.

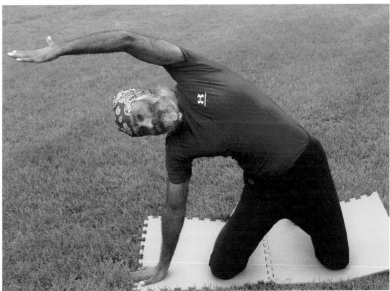 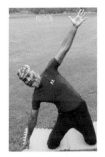

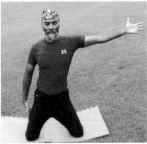

Vishram

Roll your shoulders in circles (up, back, down) about five times.
Then roll them forward (up, forward, down) five times.

REPEAT TRIKONASAN ON THE OTHER SIDE

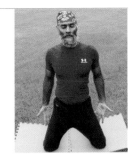

Asan: Khul & Bund Kaam Asan (open & closed core pose)

Emotional class: ਵਿਸ਼ਵਾਸ vishvaas: confidence

Physical class: ਆਧਾਰ aadhar: core strength

Mudra

This powerful pose invokes the deep abdominal muscles. Sit with legs extended so the feet are shoulder-width apart and the rope falls at or beyond the knees. You may sit on a folded blanket for back support.
Hold each rope in each hand (arms extended) shoulder height or lower. Pull down on the ropes, keeping the back as straight as possible. Squeeze the buttocks. Feel the tension in the upper abdominals.

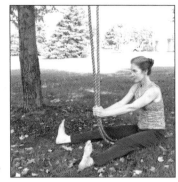

Asan

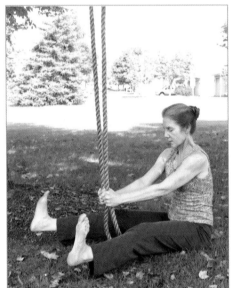

Slowly lift up the legs without leaning back. (do not make a rushed movement).
Feel strain in the groin and lower abdominals.
The feet are 4-6 inches above ground and the legs have a minimal bend at the knees.
Breath deeply and exhale forcefully, squeezing the abdominal muscles.
Hold for three breaths.

Bring the soles of the feet together towards your body. Hold onto your toes and gently stretch your knees towards the floor. Rest.

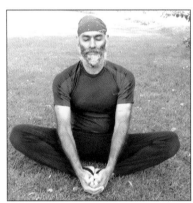

Vishram

For Khul, keep legs separated.
For Bund, keep legs together.

The core muscles are
critical for
our posture,
digestive system, and
sexual system

WITH YOGA TREE:
(alternate kaam asan)
Wrap the ropes around the outside of the tree and take each rope in each hand, pulling the ropes towards each other. Hold for three deep breaths.

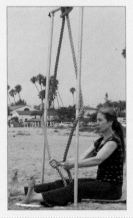

with Yoga Tree

Langar Asan (anchor pose)

Emotional class: ਏਕਤਾ ekta: oneness, harmony

Physical class: ਸਹਜ sehej: balance, poise

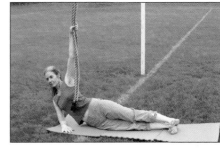

Mudra

Lie on your right side so the ropes fall at your left hip. Prop yourself up with your right elbow.
Stretch your left arm upward and hold the ropes together.
Lift your chest, keep your shoulders pressed back.
Tighten the thighs, flex the feet and engage the abdominals.

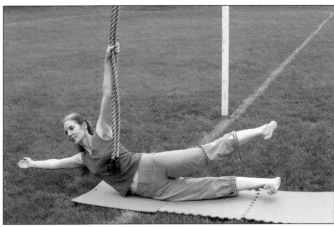

Asan

Lift both legs, left leg high.
Keep your body in a plane, using your arms for balance.
When you feel balanced, reach your right arm overhead.
The rope and your body will form an anchor-like shape.
You will feel tension along the upper thigh (outer leg) and the inner thigh (lower leg).
Side abdominals (obliques) are working to balance the body.
Hold for three breaths.
Repeat on the other side.

with Primal Shakti Yoga Tree

WITH YOGA TREE

Lie on your side so that the rope falls at the shoulder that is higher.
Hold the ropes high, adjusting your placement if the rope is not vertical.
The rope should remain vertical throughout the asan.
Keeping the body in a plane, lift the legs, flexing the feet.
When you feel balanced, extend the lower arm overhead.
Hold for three breaths.
Repeat on the other side.

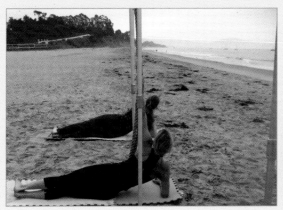

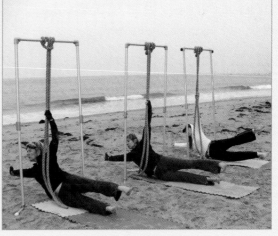

Doh Dharat Namaskar (second salute to Mother Earth)

Emotional class: ਵਾਹ wah: wonder

Physical class: ਅਨਹਦ anhad: beyond limits

Mudra

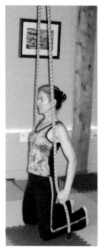

Kneel under the anchor. Take each side of the rope, one in each hand, hip high, ropes taut. Energize your triceps, shoulders, and tighten your buttocks and abdominals. Calm your mind and prepare to enjoy the asan. Bend forward at the hips, extending both arms forward, keeping legs and buttocks in vertical alignment.

Your arms are at the height of your ears.

Shift one knee toward the center for balance, curling the toes forward.

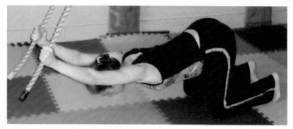

Asan

Raise and extend the other leg. Hands separated 6-12 inches. Press your chest downward. You may bend at the elbows if there is undue strain on the shoulders.

Squeeze the buttocks.

Extend arms and leg as much as possible. Feel the stretch through the abdominals as they are elongated. Try not to overarch the back.

Hold for 4 breaths.

Test your limits!

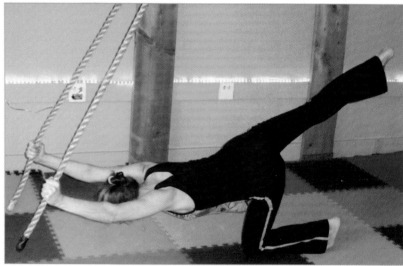

Slowly come out of the asan. Sit back and press your chest down to recover. Sway gently from side-to-side.

Repeat the asan on other side.

Vishram

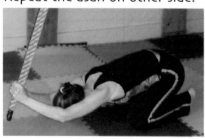

WITH YOGA TREE

First bow down, keeping one hand on the floor for balance. Other hand takes the ropes. Adjust your position so the ropes fall vertical as your body and arm is stretched while kneeling. Then take each rope in each hand and continue the asan as with the fixed anchor.

Hold for four breaths.

Repeat on the other side.

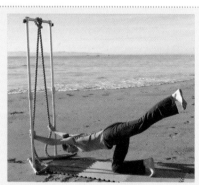

Balasan Press on Knees, Khul & Bund (strength pose)

Emotional class: विसवास vishvaas: confidence

Physical class: ਬਲ bal: strength

Mudra

Kneel a foot behind the ropes, knees apart, toes curled under, seated on your heels.

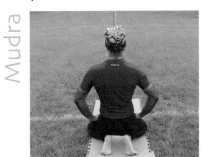

Reach forward, keeping the buttocks on the heels, and take each rope in each hand a few inches off the ground.

Keep the hands together for Bund Bal asan.

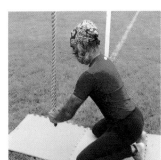

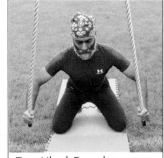

For Khul Bund asan separate the arms, keeping the elbows lifted. Pull down on the ropes, strengthening the core, shoulders, chest.

Asan

Keeping the ropes vertical and the head near the ropes, lift the knees a few inches off the ground. Be confident!

Hold for 3 breaths.

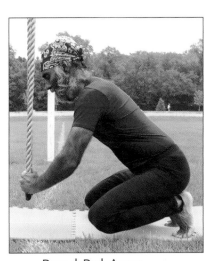

Bund Bal Asan

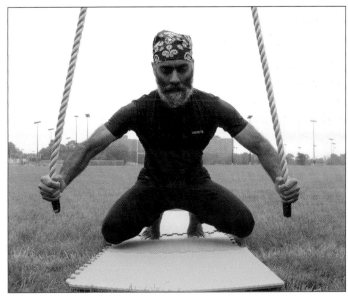

Khul Bal Asan

Vishram

Bring the knees back to the ground.
Release the ropes and stretch the arms and torso, taking a deep breath.

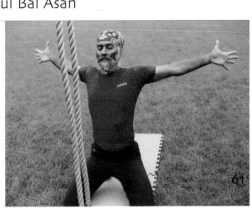

61

Hath Kaam Asan (finger press core)

Emotional class: ਵਿਸ਼ਵਾਸ vishvaas: confidence

Physical class: ਆਧਾਰ aadhar: foundation

Mudra

Sit tall with legs extended forward.
Raise the arms and extend the fingers.
Place the fingers on either side of the knees
and press the fingers into the ground.

Bend the knees slightly.
Engage the core.
Strengthen the chest and arms.
Press the feet together.

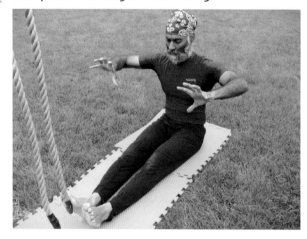
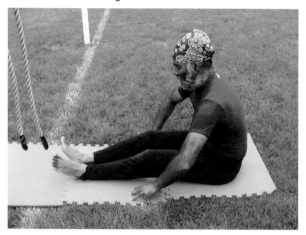

Asan

Continue pressing the fingers
and lift the legs without leaning
back, feet pressed together.
Bend the knees if you need to.
Feel confident even if your
muscles are trembling!
Hold for 3 breaths.

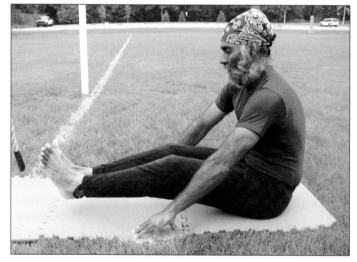

Vishram

Release.
Bring your feet towards you, bottoms of the feet
touching.
Gently hold your toes and press your knees towards
the floor, gently stretching the hips and thighs.
Take 3 shant breaths.

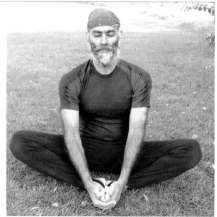

Savaar Asan (rider pose)

Emotional class: विश्वास vishvaas: confidence

Physical class: ਬਲ bal: strength

About 2 feet behind the rope, squat and sit on your heels, toes curled under (if comfortable) so the ropes are just beyond your grasp. Reach forward and take one rope in each hand.
Arms are at chest level and shoulder--width apart.

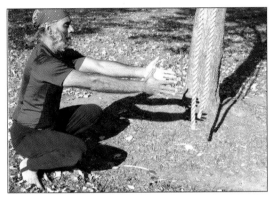 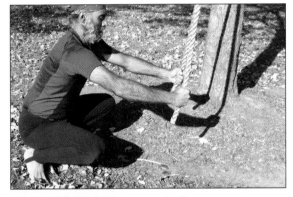

Press down on your toes and slowly press yourself off so your hips are about 2 feet off the ground. You are leaning forward with elbows bent and ropes are vertical. Feel like you are a jockey.
Hold for 3 breaths.

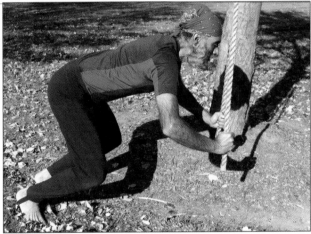

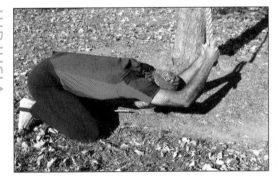

Lower yourself and press your chest down, stretching. Sway back and forth.

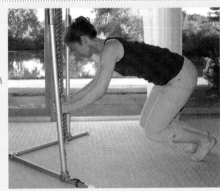

WITH YOGA TREE
Ensure that the ropes remain vertical before lifting the knees.
When you come out of the pose, do not pull the ropes toward you.

Balasan Pull (on knees) (kneeling strength pose)

Emotional class: विश्वास vishvaas: confidence

Physical class: ਬਲ bal: strength

Mudra

Kneel with your knees shoulder-width apart and bottom of the toes pressed into the floor.
Hold the ropes a few inches above your head.
Strengthen your biceps and upper body, press your toes down.
Engage your core.

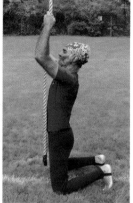

Asan

Pull your body up so your upper arms are horizontal.
Try not to pull yourself back (keep your torso vertical).
Prevent the shoulders from rising toward the ears.
Keep the abdominals and buttocks tight.
Hold for 3 breaths.

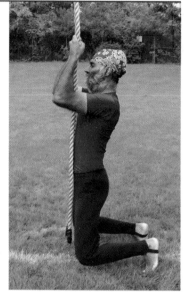

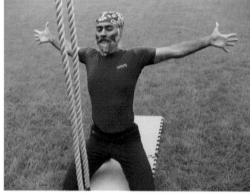

Vishram

Do a stretch opening your chest and arms and stretch the back.

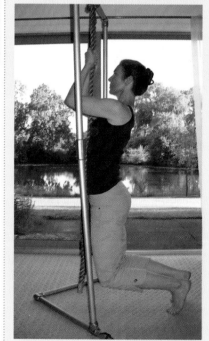

WITH YOGA TREE
Same as with anchor. Lift yourself up gracefully.

with Primal Shakti Yoga Tree

Parvat Asan (mountain peak pose)

Emotional class: ਖੋਜ khoj: explore

Physical class: ਅਨਹਦ anhad: beyond limit

Mudra

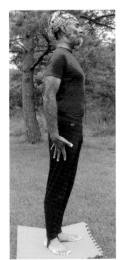

Stand in Tadasan.
Reach your arms forward and interlace the fingers.
Press your palms outward.
Keeping the arms straight, slowly raise the arms above your head.
Press your hands up, stretching your arms so they press against your ears.
Keep the chest lifted.

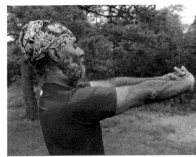

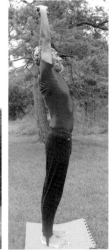

Asan

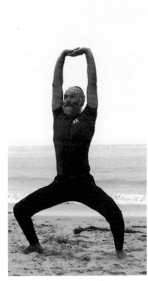

Separate your legs, adjust your feet, and come into a deep squat, continuing to lift the arms.
This is an asan of trust.
Feel truly open.
Close your eyes if you feel balanced.
Hold for three breaths.

Vishram

Release.
Open your hands and slowly make a wide circle as you lower your arms.

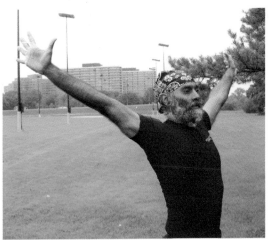

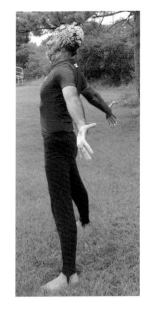

Abhay (fearless)

Emotional class: ਵਾਹ wah: wonder

Physical class: ਬਲ bal: strength

Mudra

Asan

Vishram

Take a strong stance with your feet shoulder-width apart. Press your toes and heels down as if you are planted in the ground. Hold the ropes low with elbows just a little bent. Pull your shoulder back and down. Strengthen your thighs, buttocks, core, and pull downward on the ropes. Look forward with your mind full of confidence.

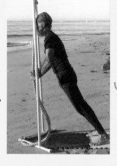

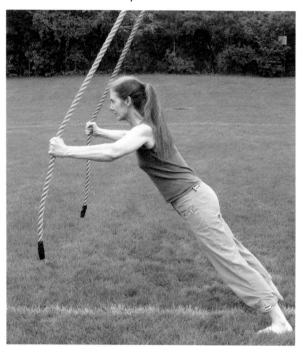

Begin leaning forward without bending at your waist, bringing your arms forward. Come forward until your hands are at eye level. Engage the core.
Hold for 4 breaths.

YOGA TREE

Stand back a few feet from the tree. Take one step forward. Take the ropes waist high, keeping them vertical. Slowly step back, keeping the body straight. Feel strain in your arms, chest and abdominal column.

with Yoga Tree

ALTERNATE STRETCH WITH YOGA TREE

Stand 1-2 feet in front of the ropes. Reach back and take both ropes in your hands at the waist. Separate the legs, taking a wide stance. With arms stretched back, lift the chest and begin squatting. Go as deep as you can, taking care not to pull the ropes toward you.
Take 1-2 breaths.

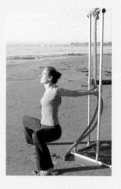

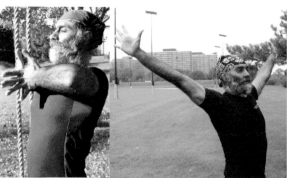

Return to a tall standing posture and press your fingers into each other, relieving the strain in your fingers, for one full breath. Then pull your arms back, stretching yourself. Close your eyes and visualize yourself soaring through the clouds. Take 2-3 breaths.

Ek Veer Asan (first warrior pose)

Emotional class: ਵਿਸ਼ਵਾਸ vishvaas: confidence

Physical class: ਅਨਹਦ anhad: beyond bound

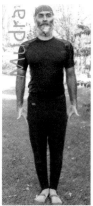 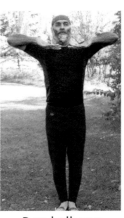 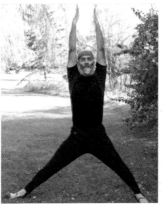 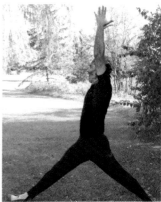

| Tadasan | Arms forward | Bend elbows | Wide stance, arms up | Twist to right |

Asan

Stand in Tadasan.
Reach the arms forward, feeling the stretch in your shoulders.
Bring your palms in toward your chest, energizing.
Either step or jump into a wide stance, so the ankles are the same distance apart as the wrists, arms extended.
Turn the right foot to the right, left foot at an angle toward the body.
Raise both arms up, palms facing.
Twist the body to the right.
Keeping the torso tall, bend the right knee, lowering the hips.
Left leg straight, buttocks tight.
Look up at the hands.
Whole body is engaged and stretched.
Hold for 3 breaths.
Release.
Repeat on the other side.

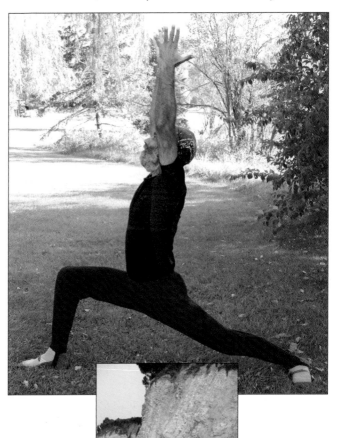

Vishram

Stand and stretch your arms, inhaling. Exhale and bring the palms together.

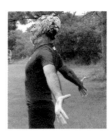

Jhoola Asan (swing pose)

Emotional class: ਸਹਜ sehej: balance, poise

Physical class: ਬਲ bal: strength

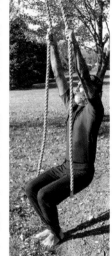
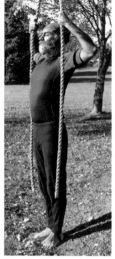

Stand under the anchor and hold (or wrap) the ropes so your hands are forehead level (you may need to find the most appropriate position with some trial). Strengthen yourself mentally and physically. Lower your hips and sit (as if in a swing). Your thighs are horizontal to the ground and your arms straight.

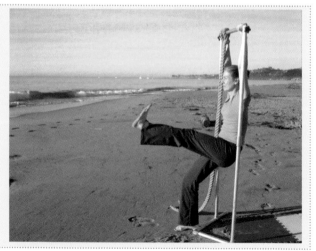

Once in the "seated" position, balance yourself by shifting the left foot to the center, and extend the right leg forward to a horizontal (or slightly above horizontal) position.
Pull your toes toward you, and press your heel forward.
Hold for 3 breaths.

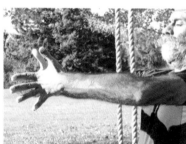
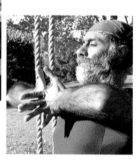

Step back and come in tadasan. Form a circle with your arms, pressing your fingers into each other. Slowly pull your hands toward your chest while inhaling. Exhale while pressing your hand forward.

YOGA TREE
Jhoola asan can be done with the yoga tree by holding the top bar of the tree, or the side bars, depending upon your height.
Then extend one foot forward and lower the hips.
Adjust your position so the tree remains vertical.

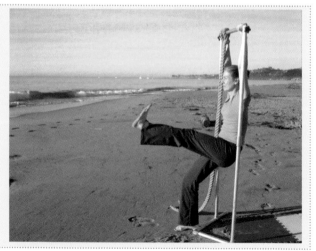

Doh Veer Asan (second warrior pose)

Emotional class: ਵਿਸ਼ਵਾਸ vishvaas: confidence

Physical class: ਅਨਹਦ anhad: beyond bound

Mudra

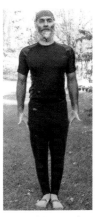
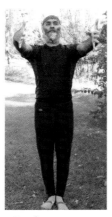
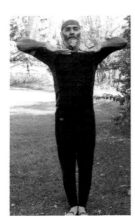
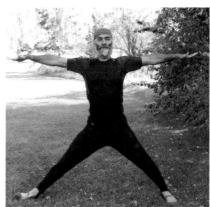

Stand in tadasan. Feel your power.
Bring your hands forward then pull them in front of your chest.
Leap (or step) into a wide stance, opening your arms into a horizontal stretch.
Spread your arms, pull your shoulders back and lift your chest.
Turn your right foot to the right side, left foot forward.
Tighten your thighs and buttocks. (see ek veer asan, page 67)

Asan

Strengthen the thighs, buttocks, lift the chest, and feel the stretch through the shoulders.
Keeping the torso tall, bend the right knee, pressing the hip down.
Keeping the arms stretched, gaze at your right arm.

Hold for 3 breaths.

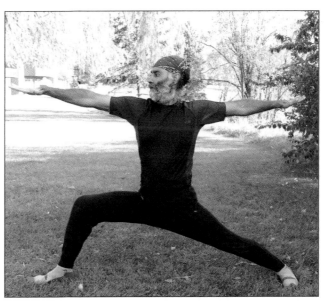

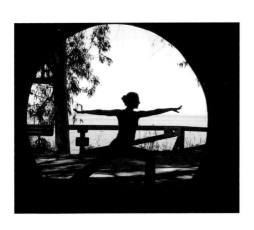

Come into tadasan and roll your shoulders in circles 3 or 4 times. Reverse the roll. Repeat Do Veer Asan on the other side.

Vishram

Chakar Asan with ropes (wheel pose with ropes)

Emotional class: ਖੋਜ khoj: explore

Physical class: ਸਹਜ sehej: balance, poise

Mudra

Stand more than arm length away from the ropes.
Lean towards the ropes to take them in your left hand.
Hold the ropes at the waist.
Calm your mind and relax.
Turn your left foot toward the left and slowly lean to the left and raise your straightened right leg so it is horizontal to the floor.

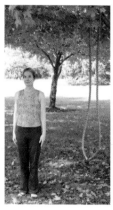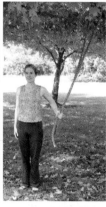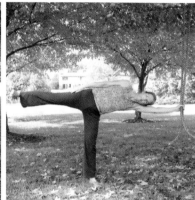

Asan

Raise your right arm vertical.
Pull your right shoulder back, lower your head so it is horizontal.
Hold for 3 breaths.
Focus your drishti on a fixed point.
Hold for three breaths.
Slowly return.

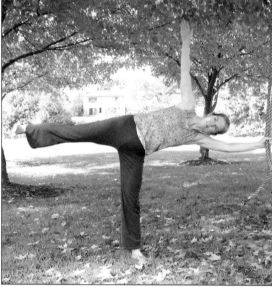

Primal Shakti Yoga Tree

WITH YOGA TREE

Stand at a distance from the Tree, so as you lean to the side, you will not be placing the rope beyond the base of the tree.
Turn out the standing foot. Continue the asan as you would with a fixed anchor.

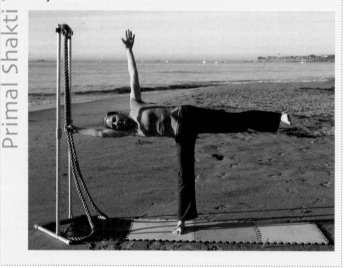

Stand in tadasan and close your eyes.
Repeat on the other side.

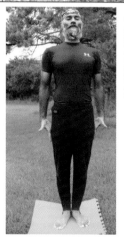

Vishram

Tricon Asan (triangle pose)

Emotional class: ਖੋਜ khoj: explore

Physical class: ਅਨਹਦ anhad: beyond bound

Mudra

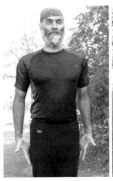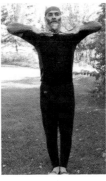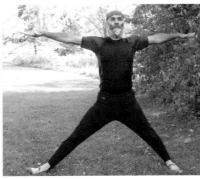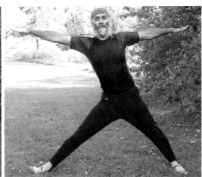

In Tadasan prepare your mind to explore your limits. Bring your hands forward and then pull them in front of your chest with forearms horizontal, chest lifted.
Feel energized. Leap into a wide stance while extending your arms horizontally.
Turn your right foot towards your right, left foot inward. Strengthen your thighs and buttocks and, keeping your legs straight, slowly reach towards your right side.

Asan

Continue bending to the right, keeping your arms stretched until either you can place your right hand on the floor, or on your leg. Keep the shoulders pressed back.
If comfortable, turn your head and look at your left hand which is pointing upward.
Hold for 3 breaths.

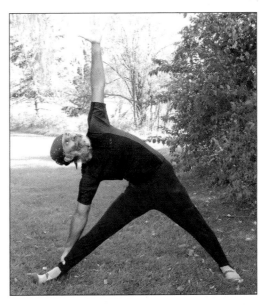

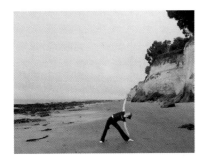

Vishram

Slowly bring your left arm down and put your hands on the floor. Bend your right knee and press your hips down, stretching.
Hold for 15-20 seconds and then bring your left foot to the right and slowly stand up.
Repeat on the other side.

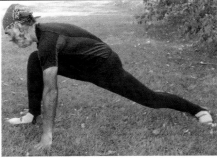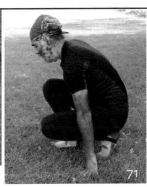

71

Bal Asan, standing (standing strength pose)

Emotional class: विश्वास vishvaas: confidence

Physical class: ਬਲ bal: strength

Mudra

Fill your mind with confidence. Take each rope in each hand at your lower abdominal level. Place the left foot under the ropes (ropes are vertical) and right foot back about 18 inches. Turn the right foot out. Bend your left knee and lean forward so your head is at the ropes. Right leg is straight and strong. Pull down on the ropes and lower your shoulders, looking forward.

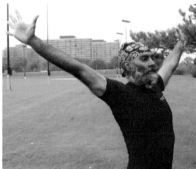

Asan

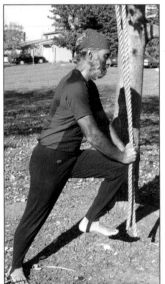

Draw your core strength and pull your left knee up touching your hands. Pull up your toes. You are leaning forward a little to build up the stress of the asan. Hold for three breaths then step down.

Vishram

Step back. Press your fingers into each other, lift your elbows, open your chest. Hold for one breath. Then pull your arms back and stretch.
Repeat the asan on the other side.

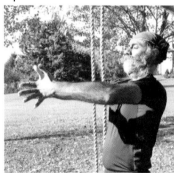

Primal Shakti Yoga Tree

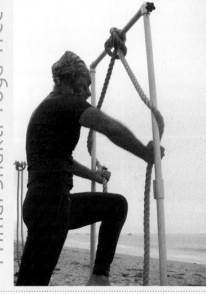

VARIATION WITH YOGA TREE
In addition to the Balasan described above, you can do this asan with the yoga tree.
Wrap the ropes around the sides of the tree and hold them with your hands a foot apart at your lower chest level. Press your shoulders down and lift your elbows. Move your right foot back about a foot from the ropes with your left foot bent at the knee and near the ropes. Strengthen your muscles and pull your left knee up. Strongly pull your hands towards each other and downward.
Hold for 3 breaths.
Release by placing your left foot down.
Repeat on the other side.

Teen Dharat Namaskar (third salute to Mother Earth)

Emotional class: ਵਾਹ *wah: wonder*

Physical class: ਅਨਹਦ *anhad: beyond bound*

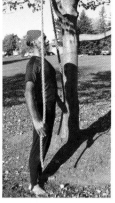
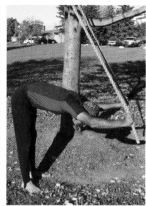

Mudra

Stand below the anchor. Hold the ropes, arms are fully extended downward. Pull your shoulders back and down, opening your chest. Strengthen your thighs and buttocks.
Lean forward, bending at the hips, extending the arms forward until you feel an optimum stretch on the upper body (chest, shoulders, arms).
Shift one leg slightly to bring it below the anchor.

Asan

Lift the other leg off the ground behind you, extending the leg, tightening the thigh (with only a small bend at the knee). You may stay with your heel on the floor, or once your balance is reached, lift up on your toes, tightening the thigh and calf muscles of the standing leg.
  Squeeze the buttocks, extend the upper body, expanding the rib cage, and tightening the stomach muscles.
Hold for four breaths.
Repeat on the other side.

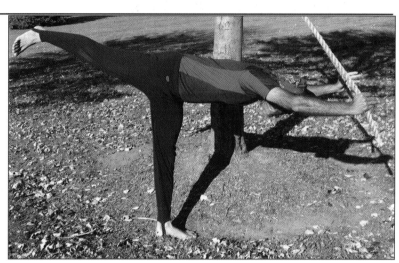

Yoga Tree

WITH PRIMAL SHAKTI
Begin by standing away from the ropes. Bend forward and step one leg forward. Take both ropes in one hand, and while bending, step back until the ropes are vertical. You may use the sides of the tree to guide your hands until you feel balanced. Continue the asan as described above.

Vishram

Step back. Press your fingers into each other.
Stretch your arms back.
Turn your hands slowly at the wrist, stretching the fingers.

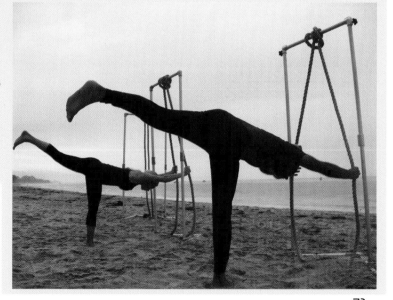

Garurh Asan (eagle pose/twist)

Emotional class: ਖੋਜ khoj: explore

Physical class: ਅਨਹਦ anhad: beyond bound

Mudra

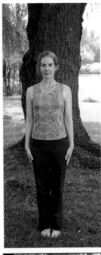 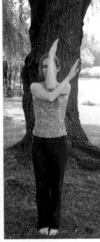 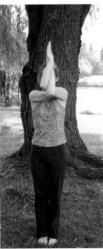

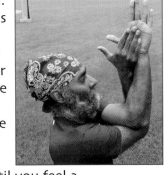

Stand in Tadasan. Extend your arms forward. Place one elbow in the bend of the other elbow. "Wrap" the outside arm around. Bring the palms together. Raise your bent arms upward until you feel a stretch across your back and shoulders.

Asan

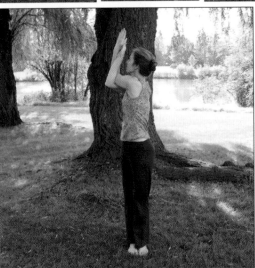 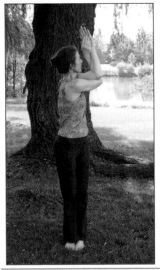

Hold the Garurh asan and slowly twist your torso as far as you can to the right.
Hold for 2 breaths, crunching the abs on the exhale.
Then slowly twist to the left.
Hold for 2 breaths. Repeat on the other side.

Vishram

"Unwrap" your arms and pull them back, opening your chest.

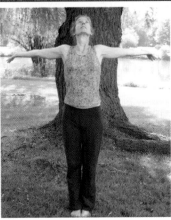

Alternate Stretch
Stand tall pressing the forearms together, raising the elbows. Slowly twist to the right.
Hold for 2 breaths, crunching the abs on the exhale.
Then slowly twist to the left.
Hold for 2 breaths.

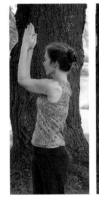 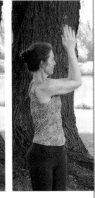

Ek Veer Asan with ropes (warrior one with ropes)

Emotional class: ਵਿਸ਼ਵਾਸ vishvaas: confidence

Physical class: ਅਨਹਦ anhad: beyond bound

Mudra

Stand tall under the anchor, holding the ropes above the head. Step forward with the left foot, toes pointing forward. Take two steps back with the right foot and turn the right foot out. Keep the shoulders and hips squared (facing forward).
Keep the chest lifted.

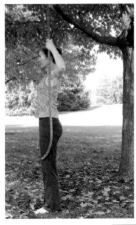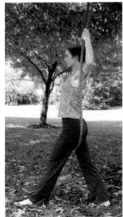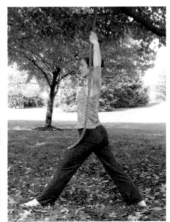

Asan

Slowly bend the left knee, pressing the hip down, sliding the hands down the rope to accommodate your stretch.
Feel the stretch in the legs and torso.
Hold for 3 breaths.

Primal Shakti Tree

YOGA TREE
same as with fixed anchor.
Final stretch (see below) is done by keeping the elbows bent and rope vertical. Or you may hold onto the bars of the yoga tree.

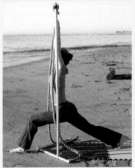

Vishram

Slowly straighten the leg, lift the chest. Then lower the hands down the rope to waist-high. With legs straight, begin reaching the torso forward and lower the torso gently. Take shant breaths as you relax into the stretch. Repeat on the other side.

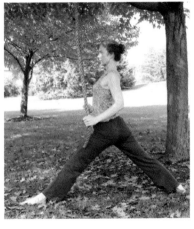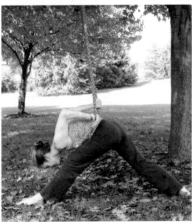

Ulta Bahar & Antar Kaam Asan (upside-down core poses)

Emotional class: ਵਿਸ਼੍ਵਾਸ vishvaas: confidence

Physical class: ਆਧਾਰ adhar: foundation

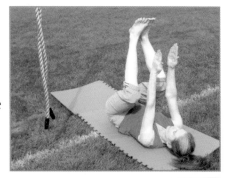

Mudra

Lie on your back. Keep the ropes aside; you do not need them for this asan. Lift and separate both knees, shoulder-width apart, about 2 to 3 feet off the ground, heels touching. Extend your arms upwards, palms facing each other, and place your forearms between the knees.

Asan

Press the arms outward against each knee using triceps and shoulders. Squeeze the knees inward, using abdominals and groin muscles. Increase the outward pressure of the palms, and the inward pressure of the knees until you feel yourself trembling. Hold for 3 breaths.

feel yourself trembling...

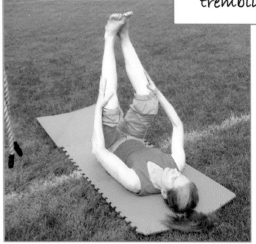

Ulta Bahar Kaam Asan
Keeping the knees lifted, press the palms (or forearms for variation) against the outside of the knees, elbows lifted. Press the arms in, press the knees out. Squeeze the buttocks, groin muscles, and feel yourself trembling. Hold for 3 breaths.

Vishram

After the three breaths, release the tension by bringing the knees into the chest and giving yourself a "hug."

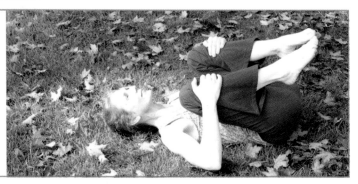

76

Seated twist (half and full)

Emotional class: ਖੋਜ khoj: explore

Physical class: ਅਨਹਦ anhad: beyond bound

Mudra

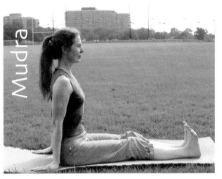 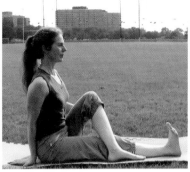 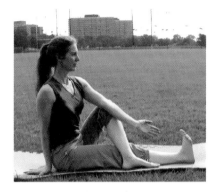

Sit tall with legs extended, palms behind you on the floor. Press your chest up. Place the left leg over the right, left foot at the right knee. Right hand is directly behind you, fingers pointed back.

Asan

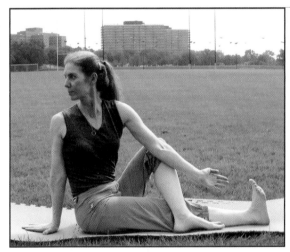

Half-twist
Swing the left arm across the left knee, straightening the arm.
Keeping the chest lifted, slowly twist the torso to look over the right shoulder. Feel the squeeze in the abdominals. Left arm is pressing the left knee to increase the stretch. Keep the chest lifted.
Hold for 3 breaths.
Repeat on the other side.

Full-twist
Place the left hand behind you.
Bring the right arm across the outside of the left knee, arm straight.
Keeping the chest lifted, slowly twist to look over the left shoulder.
Hold for 3 breaths.
Repeat on the other side.

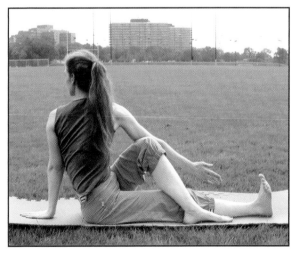

Antar & Bahar Kaam Asan (seated core)

Emotional class: ਵਿਸ਼ਵਾਸ vishvaas: confidence

Physical class: ਆਧਾਰ aadhar: foundation

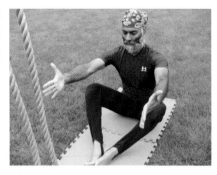

Mudra

Similar to Ulta Antar Kaam Asan (see page 76), but instead of lying down you are seated.
Lift and separate both knees, shoulder width apart, about 2 to 3 feet from your body, feet together.
Extend your arms upward, palms facing each other, and place your forearms between the knees.

Asan

Antar Kaam Asan

Press the arms against each knee using triceps and shoulders.
Squeeze the knees inward, using abdominals and groin muscles.
Increase the outward pressure of the arms, and the inward pressure of the knees until you feel yourself trembling.
Hold for 3 breaths.
Rest by bringing the feet towards the body, heels together and gently stretching.

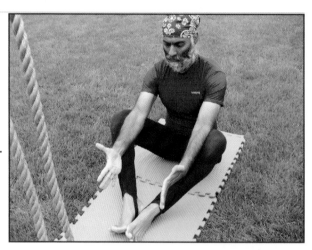

Asan

Bahar Kaam Asan

Same as Antar Kaam Asan only the palms (or forearms, for variation) are against the outside of the knees, elbows lifted.
Arms in, knees out.
Build up the pressure until you are trembling.
Hold for 3 breaths.

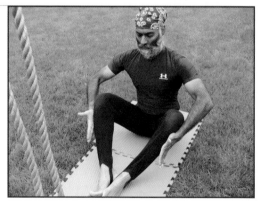

Vishram

Rest by bringing the feet towards the body, heels together. Hold the toes and gently stretch the knees out and down. Close the eyes and relax.

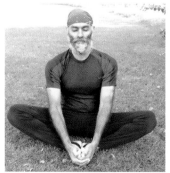

Bridge Asan (bridge pose)

Emotional class: ਏਕਤਾ *ekta: oneness, harmony*

Physical class: ਆਧਾਰ *aadhar: foundation*

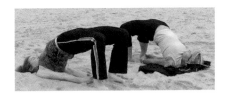

Mudra

Bridge asan opens the chest and stretches the spine. Lie on the back. Bring the feet as close to the body as possible. You may take your ankles with your hands and gently bring the feet close to your body, feet shoulder width apart and parallel. Lift the hips a bit and interlace the fingers under the hips, straightening the arms. Adjust each shoulder so they are pressed away from the ears, shoulder blades pressing towards each other.

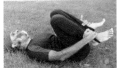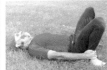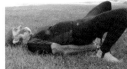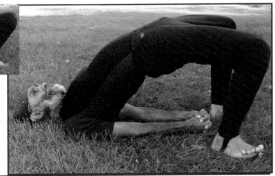

Asan

Lift the hips and squeeze the buttocks, chest reaching towards the chin. Keep the head straight. For additional intensity, pull your toes off the floor.
Hold for 3 breaths.

Lying Down Twist

Emotional class: ਏਕਤਾ *ekta: oneness, harmony*

Physical class: ਅਨਹਦ *anhad: beyond limits*

Mudra

Lie down on the back. Lift the knees into the chest, hips off the floor.
Extend the arms out to the sides of the body.
Engaging the abdominals, slowly lower both legs to the right side of the body until the legs are resting on the floor.
Use the right hand to gently press the left leg down.

Asan

Turn the head to the left, looking toward the left hand. Use shant (calm) breaths. On the exhale, feel the shoulders sinking into the floor. Feel the neck muscles relaxing. Spine lengthening.
Hold for a minute.
Repeat on the other side.

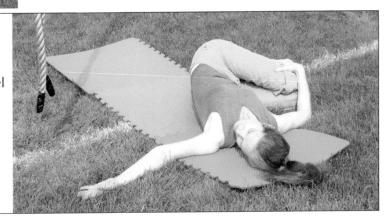

Jag Namaskar (salute to the universe)

Emotional class: ਏਕਤਾ ekta: oneness, harmony

Physical class: ਅਨਹਦ anhad: beyond limits

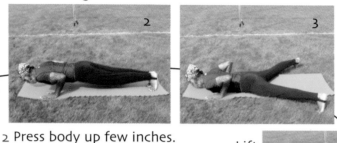

Plank position: hands next to chest, toes curled under, thighs, buttocks tight.

2 Press body up few inches. Hold for 2-3 breaths.

3 Release, widen legs.

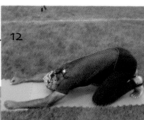

4 Lift chest, straighten arms

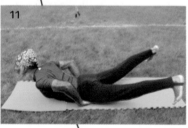

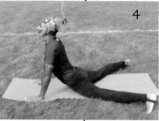

5 Press hips up, head between arms, back straight. Hold for 2-3 breaths

12 Release and rest in child's pose.

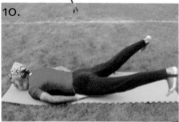

11 Lift chest, press elbows back, look ahead. Hold for 1-2 breaths.

6 Turn hands in, fingers facing inward.

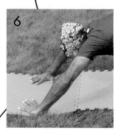

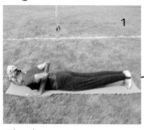

10 Tighten buttocks, thighs, lift legs, feet flexed.

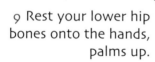

7 Lower torso, head just off the floor, elbows bent. Hold for 2-3 breaths.

9 Rest your lower hip bones onto the hands, palms up.

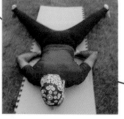

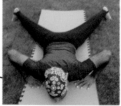

8 Slowly lower yourself to the floor

80

Agni Lapat (flame of fire)

Emotional class: विश्वास vishvaas: confidence, ਵਾਹ wah: wonder

Physical class: ਬਲ bal: strength

Mudra

Sit under the anchor. Take each rope in each hand, just above the shoulders. Lie back. Adjust the feet so they are more than shoulder-width

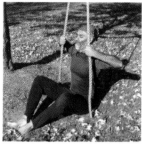 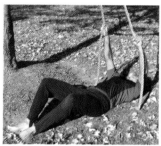 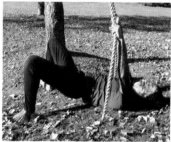

apart, with the feet pressed firmly into the floor. Focus on the anchor. Strengthen the thighs, buttocks. Start lifting the hips.

Asan

Pull on the ropes, lifting the chest, elbows out to the sides. Upper arms are in a line. Do not turn the wrists. Lift the chest as you inhale, feeling strong and confident. Keep the buttocks squeezed. You may lift the toes up, pressing the heels into the floor.
Hold for 3-5 breaths.

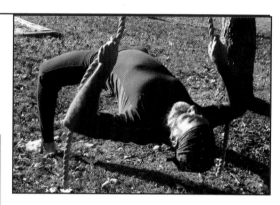

Vishram

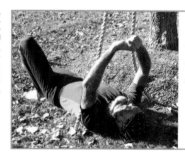

Slowly release. Massage the fingers and forearms then stretch the arms overhead.

with Primal Shakti Yoga Tree

YOGA TREE
You may wish to place a mat or blanket on the "V" portion of the Tree. Lie down before taking the ropes. Position yourself so that your shoulders are even with the side bars of the tree. This will ensure maximum stability. Bring the feet to the floor, more than shoulder-width apart, close to the body. Once positioned, reach the arms up and take each rope in each hand. Focus on the center of the top bar. Strengthen the thighs, squeeze the buttocks and slowly lift the hips, bringing the elbows out to the sides, just along the side bars.
Hold for 3-5 breaths.

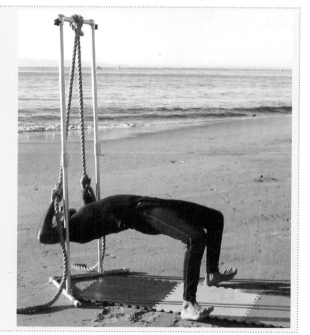

Dand Agni Lapat (flame of fire, body straight)

Emotional class: ਵਿਸ਼ਵਾਸ vishvaas: confidence, ਵਾਹ wah: wonder

Physical class: ਬਲ bal: strength

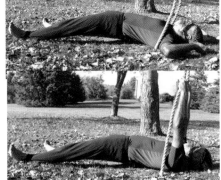

Mudra
Lie under the anchor with the ropes falling at the shoulders. Body is straight. Feet separated. Press the heels into the floor. Begin to lift the hips, feeling the strength in the thighs and buttocks. Reach the arms up and take each rope in each hand. Infuse yourself with confidence and wonder.

Asan
Focus on the anchor. Lift the body up, elbows out to the sides. (you may also tuck the elbows into the body). Lift as high as you can, aiming for the upper arms to form a line. Keep buttocks and thighs tight.
Hold for 3-5 breaths.

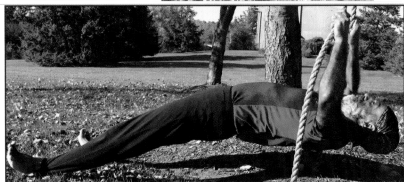

Vishram
Slowly release. Massage the fingers and forearms then stretch the arms overhead.

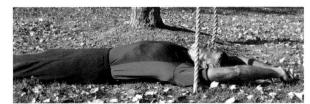

Primal Shakti Yoga Tree
YOGA TREE
You may wish to place a mat or blanket on the "V" portion of the Tree. Lie down before taking the ropes. Position yourself so that your shoulders are even with the side bars of the tree. This will ensure maximum stability. Body straight, heels pressed into the floor. Once positioned, reach the arms up and take each rope in each hand. Focus on the center of the top bar. Strengthen the thighs, squeeze the buttocks and slowly lift the hips, bringing the elbows out to the sides, just along the side bars. (do not tuck the elbows while using the yoga tree).
Hold for 3-5 breaths.

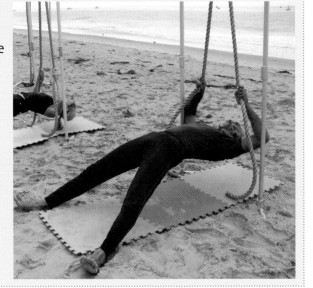

Emotional class: ਵਿਸ਼ਰਾਮ *vishram: rest*

Physical class: ਧਨਵਾਦੀ *dhanwadi: grateful*

Mudra

The yogi now prepares for the end—nirvan. The shoulder stand energizes the body and the shavasan (corpse pose) relaxes it. The yogi has recognized—after all the battles and conquests—that he/she is one with the Earth and the Sun. The gravity that causes his muscles to ache also allows them to grow. The gravity that causes breasts to sag and shoulders to droop can also be used to raise the chest, tighten the abdominals, and hold the body tall. The yogi is content and ready to face the world.

Asan

Shoulder Stand

Lie on the back with a folded blanket under the shoulders.
Place the palms down on the floor.
Bend the knees and bring them up toward the stomach.
Bring the hands behind the back and lift the hips so the knees are reaching overhead.
Raise the legs straight up.
You may support your hips with your hands or leave the arms flat on the floor, whichever is more comfortable.
The legs should be together and the toes pointed up.
Keep the head straight.
The chin should be pressed against the chest.
Breath gently through the nostrils while the posture is held.

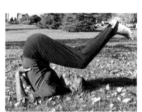

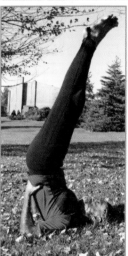

Asan

Halasan (legs overhead)

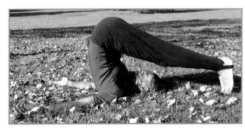

Slowly bend the knees toward the head.
Straighten the legs overhead as far as comfortable.
If possible, touch the toes to the floor.

Vishram

Shavasan (corpse pose)

Give up all control!

> Rise up, renewed, energized, light in body and mind!

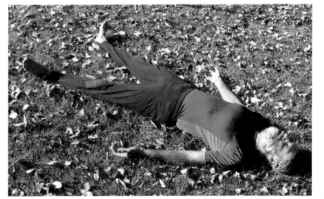

Necessity may be the mother of invention,
but play is certainly the father.

-Roger von Oech
President, Creative Think

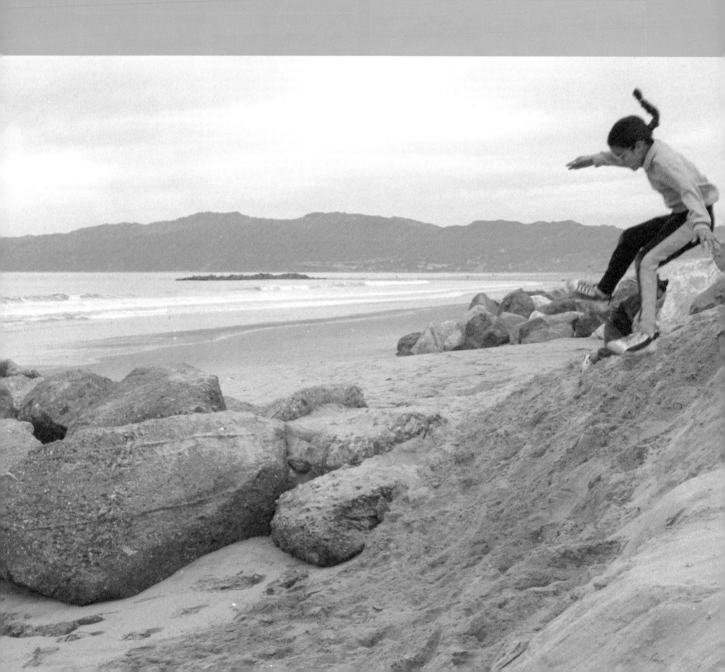

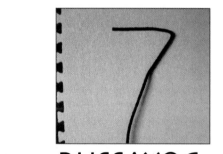

RUSSAYOG:
YOUTH CLASS SEQUENCE

Physical fitness is a critical part of a child's development. Not only is a fit body good for health, it is also good for emotional well-being. Participation in sports is one way to get fit. However, the competitive nature of sports is not suited for all youth. Additionally, sports can produce undue stress—both physical and mental—due to the win-lose nature of the game. Traditional yoga, while very good for youth, can be too slow-paced for young minds. It is difficult for teens to silently go through pranayama and asans. Russayog offers an ideal mind-body fitness program for young people. It builds long, strong muscles, a flexible body with a powerful core, and a calm mind that can focus. The RussaYog program described below will not only build a strong body, it will also help youth learn to focus and dissipate negative aspects of stress.

A fixed anchor is necessary for most bal-lila and asans which use the rope, although the bal-lila and asans can be modified while using the Primal Shakti® Yoga Tree.

Introduction: (~2 minutes)

The class begins with a 2-minute description of yogic breathing ie., low breathing, pressing the belly out and inhaling up and then exhaling downward. Essentials include the importance of stretching (lengthening the muscles and improving flexibility), strength building, balance, and mental calmness.

Free Play: (~3 minutes)

The students can do 3 minutes of free play using the ropes to stretch, sway, jump, and swing (carefully). The free play will get some of the muscles ready.

Pranayam-Breathwork

The basic pranayam sequence used for children are the Shant breath and the Jaag breath. It is easy for youth to follow these sequences.

Basics of the Yogic Breath

ਸ਼ਾਂਤੀ 1. Shanti (Peace)

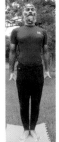

Sit in Sukhasan or standing in a relaxed state.
Take 3 breaths
through the nose.
Close your eyes.
Visualize being in harmony.

ਜਾਗ 2. Jaag (Awaken)

Visualize yourself awakening to a beautiful moment like sunrise, springtime, a flower. Stand in Tadasan with hands pressed together in front of the navel. Inhale and open your arms sideways and upwards reaching up high. Exhale bringing your arms downward and go into the Namaskar position with hands folded in front of your chest.
Inhale once in this folded hand position. Exhale and bring your arms back down opening your chest.

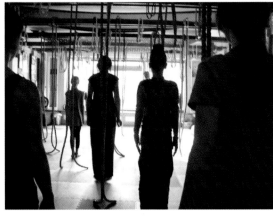

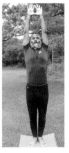
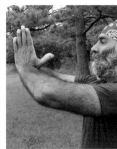
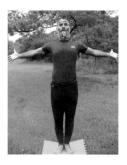

Chakars: Bal-lila and Veer-lila

The youth program involves a series of chakars, or rounds, each lasting 3-4 minutes. A chakar is made up of bal-lila (aerobic movements–with and without ropes), a pranayam (breathing sequence), vishram (rest), and an asan. One can mix and match the sequences from one session to the next to add variety. The sequences are chosen to strengthen and lengthen all muscles and develop balance and coordination. The use of ropes makes the movements fun and at the same time very empowering.

Bal-lila

Pull-ups-squats

Take the ropes, one in each hand, at your face level.
Step back and take a wide stance.
Squat till your arms are stretched and then pull yourself up to the starting position.
Do about 20 repetitions.

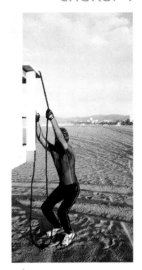

Pranayam

Step back from the ropes and press your hands into each other in front of your stomach lifting your chest.
Close your eyes and take 3 breaths.
Open your eyes and stand in Tadasan. Stand tall with your feet together, press your toes into the floor, strengthen your thighs, keeping your knees slightly bent. Tighten your buttocks. Pull your shoulders back and down opening your chest. Spread your fingers and press your hands into the sides of your thighs. Take 3 slow breaths.

Do Jaag pranayam.

Asan

Dandasan

Lie on your stomach. Place your hands by your chest and pull your elbows back towards your body. You can do this asan on your toes or your knees (easier).
Press your hands down strongly and press your torso up a few inches (about 3-4 inches) keeping your body straight.
Hold for 2 breaths.

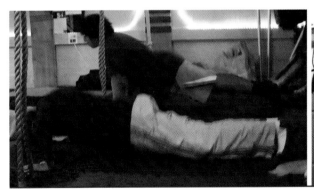
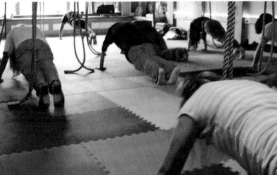

Vishram

Return to the floor and come into the child's pose. Press your hips up then sit back on your heels getting a deep stretch. You may keep your arms in front of you or by your sides.
Breathe gently, releasing any worries.

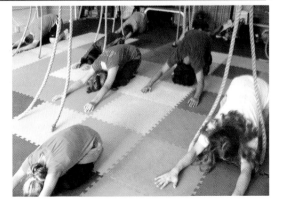

Pressdown-Squats

Take the ropes just below your waist with your arms slightly bent. Step back and take a wide stance.
Lift your chest and look forward. Squat until your hands are in front of your chest. Then press downward and raise yourself to the starting position.
Repeat 20 times.

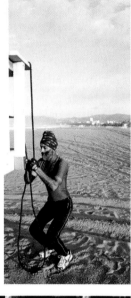

Shant and Jaag Pranayam

Repeat the pranayam sequence.

Ek Dharat Namaskar with Two Hands

Lie on your stomach holding each rope section in each hand.
Press your hands forward and hold the rope so your hands are about 6 inches above ground.
Press your feet into each other.
Strengthen your thighs and buttocks.
Pull down on the rope, lifting your chest and legs off the ground.

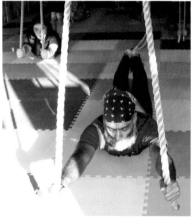

Hold for 2-3 breaths (about 25 seconds).

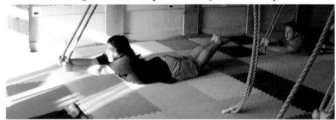

Then relax and come into the child's pose.

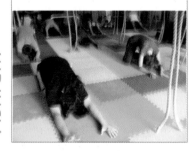

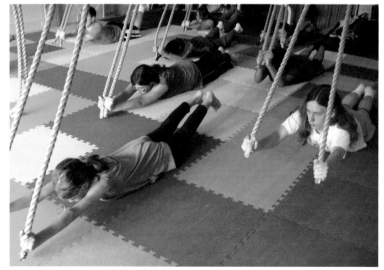

Bal-lila

Forward Lunge Stretches

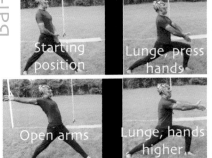
Starting position

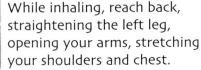
Lunge, press hands

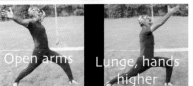
Open arms | Lunge, hands higher

Open arms | Lunge, hands higher

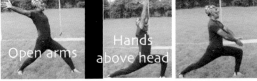
Open arms | Hands above head

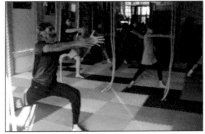

Begin with a wide stance, left foot pointing forward, right foot behind you at an angle to the right. Bend at your left knee, keeping the right leg straight.
Do not let left knee go beyond the toes.
Press your hands in tight just above the knee.

While inhaling, reach back, straightening the left leg, opening your arms, stretching your shoulders and chest.

Exhale bending your left knee, bringing your hands forward a little higher than the starting position.
Repeat, each time bringing your hands up a little higher until your hands are almost vertical.

Then continue bringing your hands downward with each lunge.
5 lunges on the left and 5 lunges on the right.

Asan

Bal Asan

Kneel tall with your feet separated about 8-12 inches behind you. The ropes are coming in front of your chest. Reach up and hold the ropes, one in each hand. Your arms are bent at a 45 degree angle. Slowly pull your body up till you are about 8 inches above ground. Hold for 2 breaths.

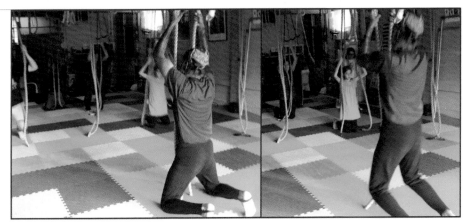

Pranayam/Vishram

Come down and stretch your chest and shoulders by holding the ropes and leaning forward while on your knees. Move a little from side to side opening, the sides of your chest.

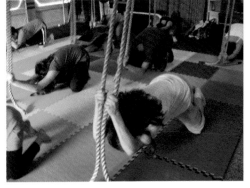

Bal-lila

Jump-floats

Hold the ropes, one in each hand, a few inches above your head so your elbows are bent. Take a shoulder-width stance with your feet. Come down so your arms are extended and push off with your toes jumping upwards. Slowly float downward so your feet make very little sound when you land.
Do your best.
Repeat for 10 jumps.

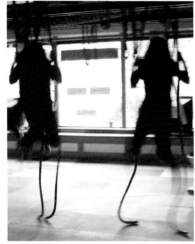

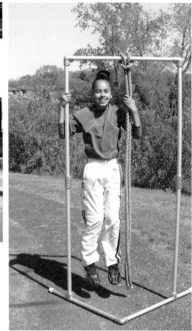

Shant and Jaag Pranayam

Repeat the pranayam sequence.

Asan

Inverted Stretch

Lie on the floor and place your hands by the side of your chest.
Open your legs wide.
Press your chest up, arching upwards.
Lift your hips up and then press your shoulders back and down without bending your legs.
Try to bring your heels on the floor.
Hold for 2 breaths.

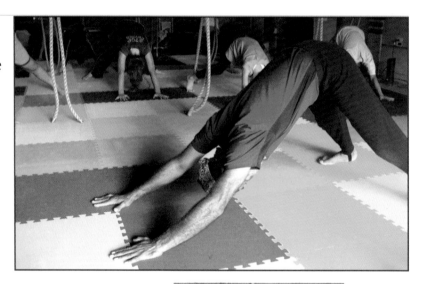

Vishram

Slowly come down and go into child's pose.

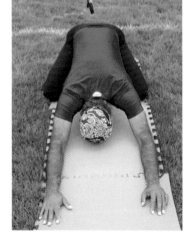

Bal-lila

Front High Kicks

Hold the ropes high, one in each hand. Balance yourself and do 10 high kicks using your right leg. Repeat on the left leg. Try to keep your legs straight and do your best.

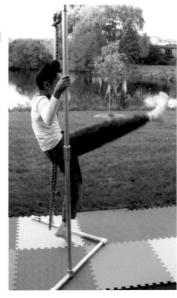

Shant and Jaag Pranayam

Repeat the pranayam sequence.

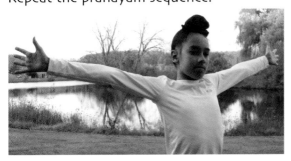

Asan

Parvat Asan

Take the tadasan position.
Now press your hands forward until they are horizontal.
Interlock your fingers and turn your hands so the palms are facing forward.

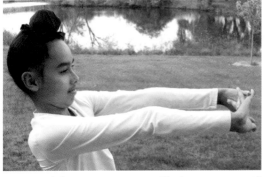

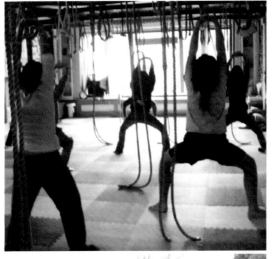

Start raising your arms till they are vertical and as straight as possible.
Take a wide stance, turing your feet outward so you are comfortable.
Squat down, keeping your chest vertical.
Go as deep as you feel like and don't go deeper than the point where your thighs are horizontal.

Hold for 2-3 breaths (about 25 seconds).

Slowly come up and inhale, opening your arms. Exhale and come into the Namaskar position. Exhale, opening your arms to the sides and stretch.

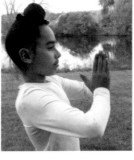

Pull-ups from the Floor

Sit under the rope anchor and hold the ropes
just above your head with each hand.
Lean back.
Straighten your legs, separating them
shoulder-width apart.
Strengthen the thighs and press your heels
into the floor, squeezing the buttocks.
Keeping your body straight, engaging the
abdominal muscles, raise your hips upward,
pulling your body up at the same time.
Do 10 repetitions.

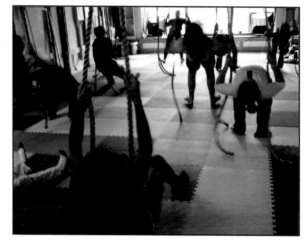

Shant and Jaag Pranayam
Repeat the pranayam sequence.

Teen Dharat Namaskar

Stand tall with the ropes by your sides.
Take the ropes low, arms straight.
Bend forward at your hips, stretching
your chest and back.
Bend your elbows if you feel undue
shoulders strain.
Bring your foot to the center.
Keep your gaze fixed on a focal point.
Slowly press your right leg back and lift
it as high as you can.
Hold for 3 breaths.

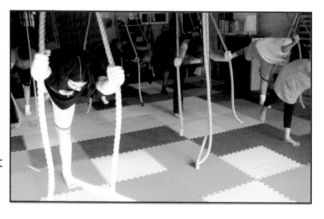

Slowly come out and stretch
with the ropes, doing any
favorite stretch.

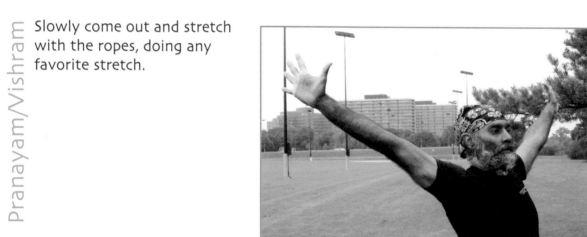

ਲਚਕ flexibility ਬਲ strength ਸ਼ਾਨ poise

Side Kicks

Bal-lila

Hold the ropes for balance. You can adjust the hold, if you need to, as you start your kicks. Stand tall and raise your leg sideways as high as you can. Try not to lower your torso too much.
Do 10 kicks on the right side
and then 10 on the left side.

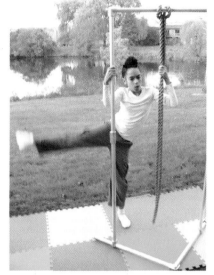

Bal Asan (Standing)

Asan

Stand and hold each rope in front of the waist.
Bring the left foot under the anchor.
Step back with the right foot, turning the foot out.
Bend the elbows out slightly.
Bend the front knee, and bring the head forward, strengthening the back leg.
Pull down on the ropes.
Lift the left leg, flexing the foot.
Engage your core by tightening the abdominal muscles as you exhale.

Hold for 3 breaths.

Slowly come down.

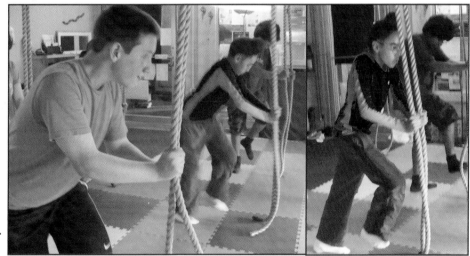

Pranayam/Vishram

Step back from the ropes and press your hands into each other in front of you, lifting your chest, elbows lifted.
On the inhale, pull your hands towards your body maintaining the inward pressure.
Exhale pressing your hands forward, then relax.

Repeat Bal Asan on the other side.

Press your hands together and breath, relieving any stress from your fingers.

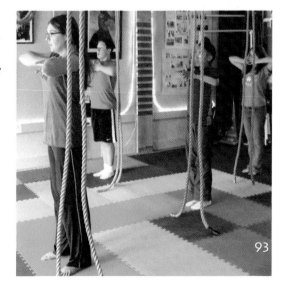

93

Chakar 8

Jump/Knee-ups

Hold the ropes above your head, elbows bent.
Squat and then jump, pulling your knees up.
Slowly float down, landing so your feet make very little sound when you land.
Do your best!
Repeat for 10 jumps.

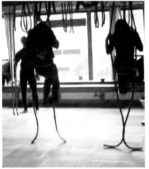

Repeat the pranayam sequence.

Doh Veer Asan

second warrior pose

Begin in Tadasan.
(see page 69)
Stay strong.
Hold for 3 breaths.

Slowly straighten the leg, face the toes and torso forward, and repeat on the other side.

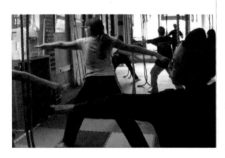

Chakar 9

Two-hand punches

Squat low, wide stance.
Make fists with your hands at your waist.
Throw your hands out, open your hands and exhale.
Rapidly bring your fists back and inhale.
10 repetitions.

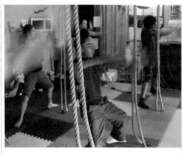

Jhoola Asan

(see page 68)

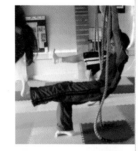

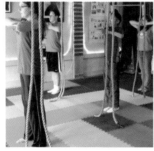

Press your hands together, inhale.
Exhale, pressing your hands back, and relax.
Repeat Jhoola Asan on the other side.
End with the same breath sequence.

Chakar 10

Arm Stretches

Kneel, hold the ropes, lean forward, inhale, while pressing your chest down.
Exhale while raising your torso.
Repeat 10 movements.

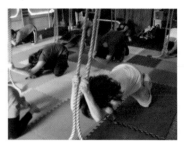

Ek Veer Asan/ Ropes

first warrior pose

See page 77
Hold for about 25 seconds.

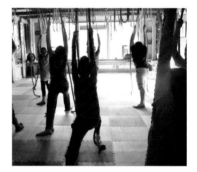

Bring your hands down the ropes to the waist, straighten the legs and stretch the torso, bringing your chest towards your thigh.
Breathe and hold 25 seconds.

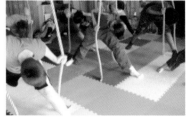

Repeat Ek Veer Asan and the Stretch on the other side.

Chakar 11

One-hand punches

Squat and punch, exhaling.
One hand at a time.
Do for 10 repetitions.
Repeat on the other side.
Close your eyes.
Take 3 breaths.

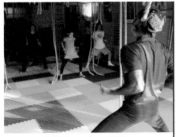

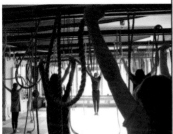

Chest Stretch/Rope

Reach overhead, keeping
the rope taught.
Slowly lower the rope
behind your head,
maintaining the pressure
on the rope. Slowly raise
the rope up again.

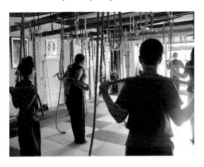

Roll your shoulders
to recover.

Chakar 12

Leg Raises

Hold the ropes & raise
your legs while exhaling.
Bring your legs down
while inhaling.
Try not to lean back.
Do 10 repetitions.

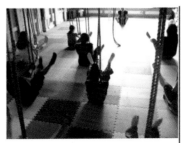

Vishram

With your hands pull
your feet toward your
body, gently press the
knees down.

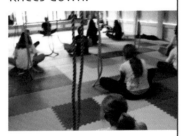

Hath Kaam Asan

Press your fingers into the
floor and lift the legs.
Take 2 breaths.

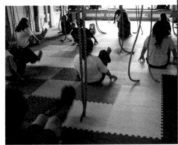

Chakar 13

Pull-ups

Sit and hold the ropes above
your head. Lean back. Press
your feet into the floor and
raise your body up.
Do 10 repetitions.

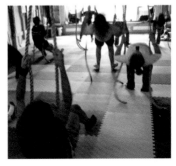

Pranayam

Release, massaging your
hands.

Lying Down Twist

Lie down, then lower your
knees towards your left
elbow. Slowly turn your head
towards your right hand,
close your eyes and relax.
Hold for about 25 seconds.
Repeat on the other side.

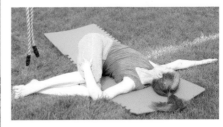

Ending:

Shavasan
Lie on your back, eyes closed.
Begin to relax. Take slow
breaths and calm your mind.
Visualize a peaceful place.
Stay in Shavasan 5-20 minutes.

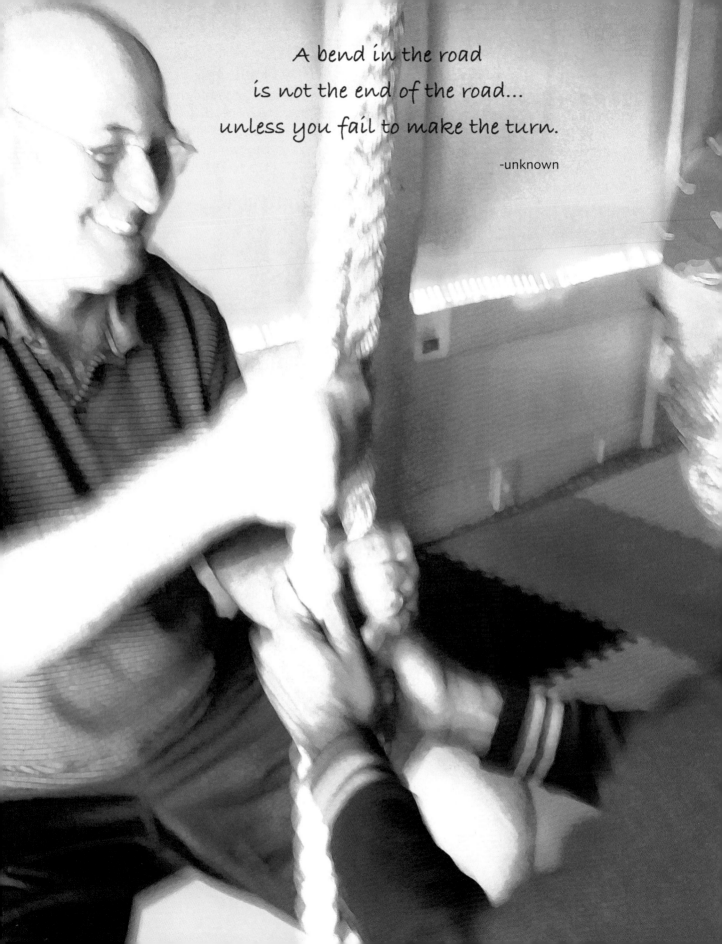

A bend in the road
is not the end of the road...
unless you fail to make the turn.

-unknown

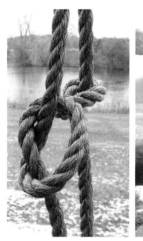
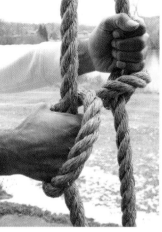

I will not ask for a
lighter burden,
but for
broader shoulders.
-Jewish proverb

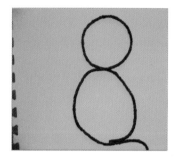

RUSSAYOG FOR PERSONS WITH LOW MOBILITY

Consider the following scenarios: As a result of a stroke, you have weakened use of your left arm and leg, but are otherwise vigorous (there are 4.7 million Americans in this situation); due to poor eating habits or due to genetic challenges you are obese (a third of the U.S. population); due to aging you are developing early signs of Parkinson's' disease (a rapidly growing segment of the population); due to an accident you are temporarily unable to use your full mobility...

The doctor's advice regarding exercise goes something like, "You should exercise as much as you can without pain. Exercise will not only improve your physical health, but it will improve your mental health." Apart from walking, which is a great exercise, what else can you do? Traditional gyms with weights, exercise cycles, stepping machines, etc., may be imposing or difficult to use. For the low-mobility population, most traditional yoga poses are daunting without props. RussaYog, with its usage of ropes, offers an excellent choice.

The ability to hold onto a rope, even if only one hand is able to hold it, immediately provides confidence to the student. While canes, crutches, walkers, etc., are very helpful for low-mobility users, ropes allow one to pull and press, balance, lengthen, and strengthen muscles. The low-mobility group could find RussaYog most beneficial.

The RussaYog workout described in Chapters 4, 5, and 6 can be customized for the benefit of low mobility users. The customization would be based in part by the physical abilities of the user.

Can you grip a rope with each hand?
Can you grip a rope with only one hand?
Can you stand while holding ropes?
Will you need to stay in a wheelchair or to have to stay seated on a bench/chair?

If a rope is difficult to grip, one can use a modified "ladder rope" made of canvas.
A specially stitched "rope" made from canvas belts can be made. The slots in the belts can allow the user to secure the hand and hold the "rope."
Here are two typical sessions:

A) for an elderly person with special needs.
B) for a stroke survivor with weakened control of the left hand.

The workouts and other similar customized workouts can be used for the elderly with special needs, obese persons, and people with various disabilities. Everyone needs to exercise and RussaYog builds confidence while providing exercise.

Session A

A 60-90 minute session. Each asan is held for 3 breaths, as tolerated.

The following pranayam can be used to rest between Bal-lila exercises and Asans:

Standing pranayam
3 shant breaths (see Chapter 4, page 34)
3 jaagya breaths (see Chapter 4, page 34)

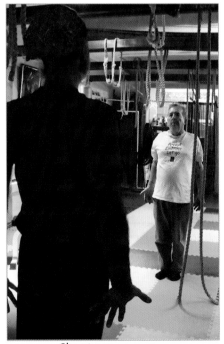

Shant pranayam

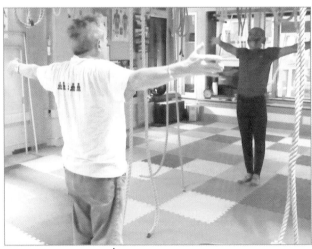

Jaagya pranayam

Start of Bal-lila
Rope pull-up squats
Do 15 comfortably

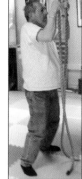
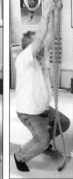

Pranayam
shant, jaagya

Rope press-down squats
(see page 40)
Pranayam

Seated Knee Lifts
Hold the ropes just above the lap, arms separated. Pull down, exhale, and lift the knees together.
Hold for a second and slowly lower them, inhaling.
Do 15 reps.

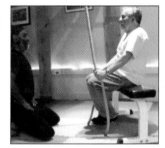

Pranayam

Seated Leg Lift
Hold the ropes in each hand waist high.
Lift right knee up and then outward, opening the hip joint.
Repeat 10 times.
Do the other side.

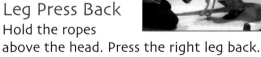

Leg Press Back
Hold the ropes above the head. Press the right leg back.
Hold for a second and bring it back, keeping the right foot off the floor.
Do 15 reps.
Stand comfortably.
Repeat on the left leg.

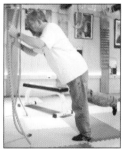

Kriya
Seated on a bench, extend the arms forward. Then inhale quickly while bringing the fists to the waist. Exhale, thrusting the arms forward, palms open.
Do 15 repetitions.

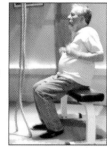

Standing Knee Lift
Pull the ropes downward and lean a little forward. Slowly lift the right knee as high as possible and then lower it.
Repeat 15 times.
Pranayam
Repeat on the other side.
Pranayam

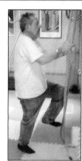

Rope Breaths
Hold one end of a rope shoulder-width apart. Pull the rope while slowly raising your arms as high as possible, inhaling. Slowly bring it down, exhaling.
Repeat 10 times.

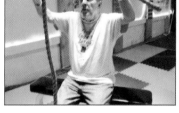

Start of Yogabhyas

Rope Pull
Hold one end of the rope with arms extended, shoulder width apart. Pull the rope to your limit.
Take 2 slow breaths.

Stretch your arms back.
Take 2 breaths.

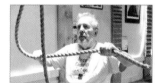

Ek Dharat Namaskar with two
hands holding the ropes. (p. 32)

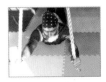

Modify the pose so you are comfortable with no pain. Pull the ropes and lift both legs. Hold for 3 breaths.

Ek Dharat Namaskar (one hand)

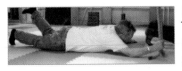

p.56
Take 3 breaths.
Rest.
Repeat other side.

Stand in Tadasan
close your eyes for 3 breaths.

Parvat Asan (p. 65)
Bend the knees if comfortable.
Pranayam: shant, jaagya

Standing Balasan
with right knee lifted. (p. 72)
Repeat with the other leg.

Seated Twist
Sit with arms pressed together. Slowly twist as far as possible to the right. Take 3 breaths. Then other side. Stretching breath.

Kaam Asan
Sit, ropes waist high. Pull down, without leaning back, lift both knees. Hold for 3 breaths.

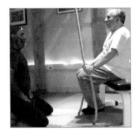

Seated Triconasan
Sit, left palm on the bench. Chest lifted. Lean to the left, bending the left elbow. Reach the right arm up slowly in a circular motion. Continue leaning as far as possible without leaning forward.

Teen Dharat Namaskar (p. 73)
The lower you hold the ropes, the more extension you will feel. Lean forward, keeping the core engaged. Lift the left leg back as high as you can.

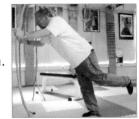

Pranayam: jaagya
Repeat on the other side.

Ek Veer Asan (p. 75)

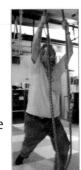

Hold the ropes high. Step forward with the right foot. Take a couple of steps back with the left foot to get a wide stance. Holding the ropes, bend the front knee. Glide the hands down the ropes. Keep the bent knee behind the toes. Hold for 3 breaths.

Jhoola Asan (p. 68)
Hold the ropes forehead level. Bend the knees as though you are sitting down. Bring the left foot to center, strengthen the buttocks, thigh, and raise the right leg. Hold for 3 breaths.

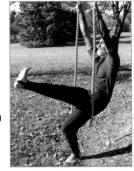

Pranayam: shant, jaagya
Repeat on the other side.

Modified Agni Lapat
Lie on the back, ropes at the shoulders. Grip the ropes as high as possible. Strengthen the core. Lift the torso, keeping buttocks on the floor. Hold for 1-3 breaths. Release.

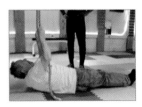

End in Shavasan.
Lie on the back, eyes closed, palms facing up. A folded blanket may be placed under the lower back for comfort. Focus on the breath. Relax the muscles.

Session B

A 60-90 minute session.

A potential session for a stroke survivor.

Pranayam is used after each movement and asan:

3 shant breaths (see page 34)

3 jaagya breaths (see page 34)

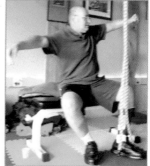

Do the session after initial therapy has been completed by a medical facility and your physician has cleared you for exercise. You can show this workout to your physician for approval.

The session is built on developing the three ingredients of recovery: strength, flexibility, and balance. The use of ropes allows one to slowly increase all three of these necessary ingredients.

Gripping the rope: Many stroke survivors may have difficulty gripping a rope due to weakness and loss of control. Several options one can use:

A trained helper can hold the rope just below the user's grip to make sure there is no slippage.

A knotted rope can be used.

The workout can be similar to the one described in Session A, ie., use seated and standing bal-lila (slowly) and asans. It is also useful to do some stretching of the arms, chest, and legs while lying on the back.

The key is to design a program that the user can perform while being challenging from the point of view of strength, balance, and flexibility. To design the program use the information given in Chapters 4, 5, and 6 and select/modify postures. Using ropes while doing knee raises builds core strength. These core muscles are otherwise difficult to exercise, since doing sit-ups and leg raises may not be options.

Pranayam

Pranayam sequence includes 3 shant breaths (standing or seated) and 3 jaagya breaths. For a stroke survivor it may be difficult to lift and extend the arms. In this case, bring the arms as high up as possible. It does not matter if the left and right sides have different control.

JUST DO YOUR BEST—and keep doing it!

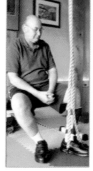

Start of Bal-lila
Rope Stretch

Hold the ropes high (as high as you can). If needed, use one hand to bring the other hand high (eg., by pulling one end of the rope using the support as a pulley). Sway back and forth and stretch your chest, shoulders, and back. Take 10 breaths as you do this.

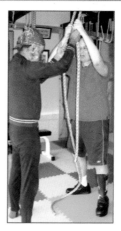

Rope pull-up squats
Hold ropes at chest.
15 done slowly.
Pranayam

Rope press-down squats
Hold ropes at waist.
15 done slowly
Pranayam

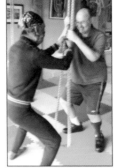

Seated on a bench/chair:
Hold the ropes above the lap. Press down, lifting the knees. Hold and slowly lower legs.
Do 15 reps.
Pranayam: shant, jaagya

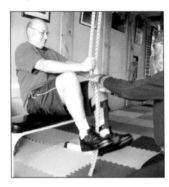

Seated on a bench/chair:
Hold the ropes above the lap. Lift one knee then move it outward, opening the hip joint.
Repeat 10 times.
Pranayam
Other leg.

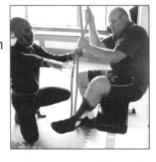

Leg Press Back
Stand tall. Hold the ropes for balance. Press the right leg back. Hold briefly.
Repeat 15 reps.
Keep the right foot off the floor.
Repeat on the other leg.

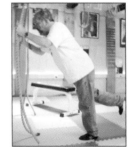

Kriya seated or standing
Extend the arms forward, inhale, bringing the fists to the waist. Exhale strongly, thrusting the arms forward, palms open. Do 15

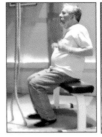
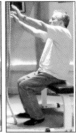

Knee lifts while standing. Hold the ropes
at a comfortable position. Pull the ropes downward and lean a little forward. Slowly lift the knee as high as possible and then lower it. Repeat 15 times.
Pranayam: shant, jaagya
Repeat on the other side.
Pranayam: shant, jaagya

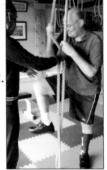

Leg lifts from prone position
Lie on the back. Lift one leg, crunching the abs. You may support your head with one hand, or both. Move the leg outward and back. Lower the leg and repeat on the other side.
10 times.

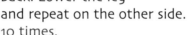
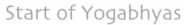

Start of Yogabhyas

Rope Pull (seated or standing)
Hold one end of the rope with arms lifted shoulder width apart. Start pulling the rope apart. Go to your limit. Don't hunch the shoulders.
Take 2 slow breaths. Stand up and take a relaxed breath.

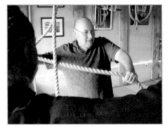

Stretch by pulling your arms back and take 2 breaths.

Ek Dharat Namaskar with two

hands holding the ropes. Modify the pose so you are comfortable and there is no pain. Pull down on the ropes and lift both legs off the ground (even if it is an inch or so). (p. 32) Hold for 3 breaths.

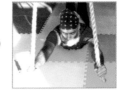

Ek Dharat
Namaskar with one hand holding
the ropes. (p. 56)

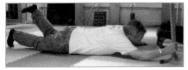

3 breaths.
Rest 3 breaths.
Other side.

Pranayam

Standing Balasan with knee

lifted and pressed to the side, foot flexed. (page 72)
3 breaths.
Pranayam
Repeat on the other side.

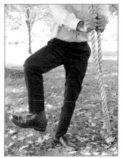

Kaam Asan

Sit on the bench. Hold the ropes in front of the waist.
Pull down on the ropes (hold a tall seated posture) and lift both knees up.
Hold for 3 breaths.

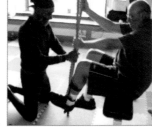

Seated Triconasan

Excellent asan to improve flexibility.
See session A. (page 100)

Standing or Seated Twist

Stand strongly with hands pressed in. Squeeze your buttocks and slowly twist as far as possible to your right, keeping your feet on the floor.
Take 3 breaths.
Return .
Twist to the other side.
Pranayam

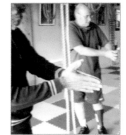

Teen Dharat Namaskar
Ek Veer Asan
Jhoola Asan
Modified Agni Lapat
See session A. (page 100)

Shoulder Press Out/In

On the back, extend the arms up. Partner will place his/her arms on the inside of the arms. Use shoulder strength and core strength to press in/partner pressing out.
3 breaths.
Repeat with arms outside, pressing out, partner pressing in.
Hold for 3 breaths.
Stretch arms overhead.

End in Shavasan. (see page 83)

optional:
Child's Pose
Close your eyes.
3 breaths.

Parvat Asan
See session A. (page 100)
At your own comfort level.

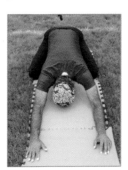

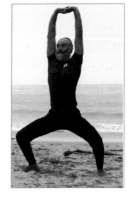

Come dear friend,
when we are face-to-face,
my body and my mind are soothed.

ਆਵੋ ਸਜਨਾ ਤੂ ਮੁਖ ਲਗ ਮੇਰਾ ਤਨ ਮਨ ਠੰਡਾ ਹੋਏ
Aao sajna Tu mukh lag mera tan man thanda hoye.

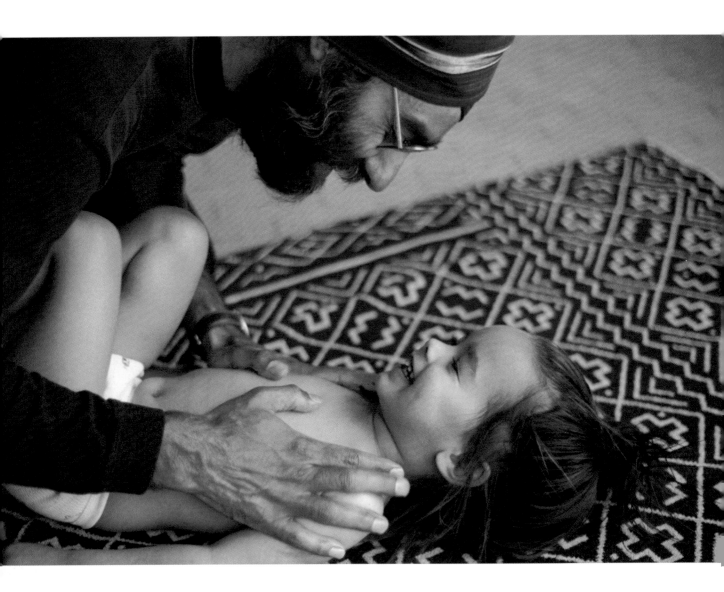

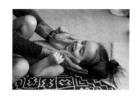

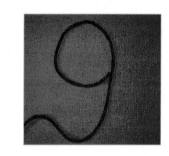

VISHRAM YOG
ਵਿਸ਼ਰਾਮ ਜੋਗ

The human body loves to be stretched and squeezed. Babies thrive when they are hugged and gently massaged. Children love to hang from bars and rings and ropes, stretching themselves. An iconic image of childhood is swinging on a rope over a pond and letting go. When we are tired we want someone to press the fatigue out of us. We hug a friend or even a stranger at time of stress or joy.

Stretching- or pressing-based massage has been part of my life since I was born. My father specialized in a massage style that lengthened muscles, opened the joints, and applied pressure to squeeze out fatigue. My mother massaged my head with her own unique style of massage. The Vishram Yoga presented here is an outcome of this tradition and developed especially for the yogi.

Vishram Yog or restful yoga involves a giver and a receiver where the giver strives to increase the flexibility of the receiver and make the receiver more self-aware. Many of the elements of Shiatsu massage can be found in Vishram Yog, although Shiatsu massage has developed more as a medical treatment. Vishram Yog is not being presented as a medical treatment—its purpose is to promote relaxation, and to increase self-awareness and flexibility.

In vishram massage the giver places the receiver's body in various stages of gentle stress and holds the pressure for about 20 seconds (about 2 breaths). There are four basic sequences:

    Receiver on back: lower body is relaxed;
    Receiver on back: arms, neck, head is relaxed;
    Receiver on stomach: lower body is relaxed; and
    Receiver on stomach: back, neck, head is relaxed.
    Additional massage can be given with the receiver seated.

Receiver should be relaxed. Giver should be tuned into the receiver's breathing.

RECEIVER ON BACK: LOWER BODY IS RELAXED

Take the right hand. Squeeze the hand gently by wrapping your hand around the fingers.
Ask the receiver to relax and not to "help" you do the massage.

With your right hand, press gently on the stomach just below the navel.
Hold for 3 breaths. With your left hand, press the stomach just below the rib cage at each of the 5 points shown. Hold each spot for about 2 breaths.

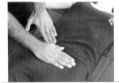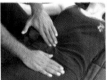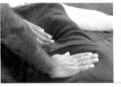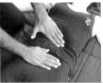

Exchange your left hand with the spot where your right hand is and use your right hand to press the upper thigh for 2 breaths. Slowly press the lower thigh, calf, and foot.

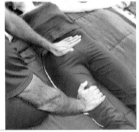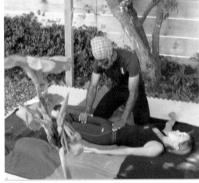

Place your left hand under the knee while holding the foot with the right hand. Lift the knee and after opening the leg outward press the knee towards the chest. Press the front of the foot down stretching the ankle joint.

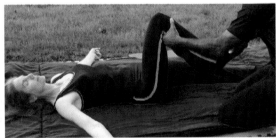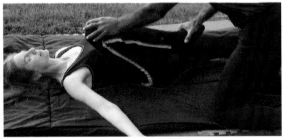

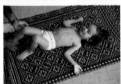

Lift the knee up and then press it down toward the side, opening the inner thighs.
Press down at a comfortable level.

Pull the knee up and place the left foot on the outside of the right knee (either with both knees bent, or with right leg straight).
Press the left knee down to the right side of the receiver.
Place your hand on the left shoulder to give a deep stretch for this twist.

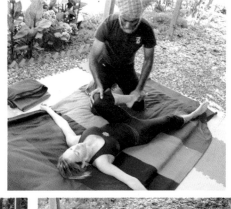

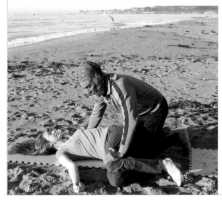

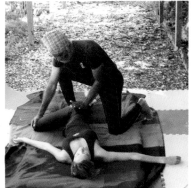

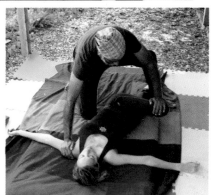

Lift the knee up, straighten the leg, and gently pull the leg.
Hold for 2 breaths.

Repeat on the other side.

Hold the ankles and bring the legs up to vertical position. Strengthen your stance and pull the legs upward. Gently move the legs, allowing the lower back to relax.

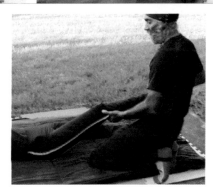

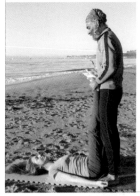

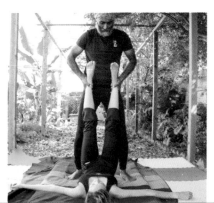

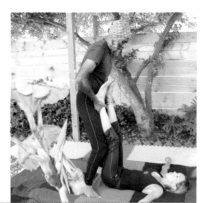

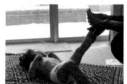

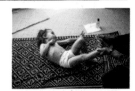

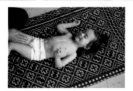

107

RECEIVER ON BACK, UPPER BODY

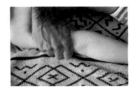

Hold the left hand with your right hand and press the forearm and upper arm. Raise the arm high, stretching the arm and shoulder.

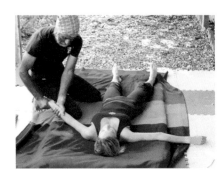

Fold the arm across the chest, pressing on the upper arm/shoulder area.

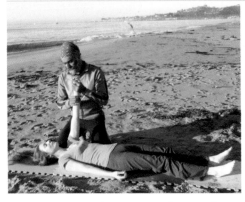
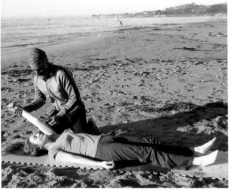
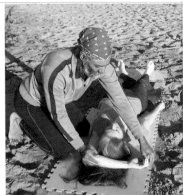

Raise the arm and stretch it overhead.
Press down on the upper arm.
Fold the arm at the elbow and press down.
Pull both arms back, stretching the back and chest.
Repeat on the other side.

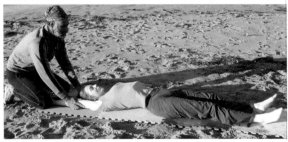

RECEIVER ON THE BACK: HEAD AND NECK

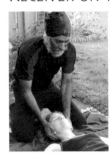

Cradle the head with both hands and gently stretch the neck.
Turn the head and gently press.
Press the temple area, various areas on the head, with the palm.
Use the fingers and thumb to massage the scalp.

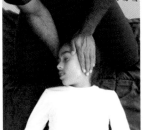
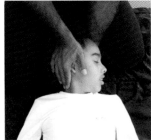

Massage the earlobe and area of the head under the ear by rubbing it.

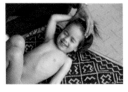

Repeat after turning the head to the right side.

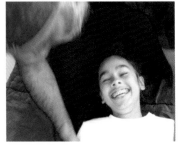

RECEIVER ON STOMACH: LOWER BODY
Press down on the lower back with right hand.

Keep the right hand pressed on the lower back, and with the left hand, apply pressure (for two breaths each) on buttock, upper thigh, lower thigh, calf.

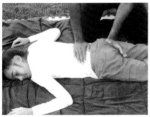 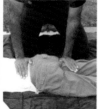 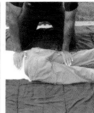 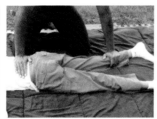 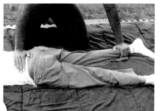

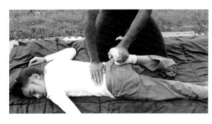

Hold the foot of the right leg and separate the leg out and bend the leg, pressing the heel of the left foot into the buttocks.
Hold the pressure for two breaths.
Bring the lower leg down and pull on the leg.

Gently hold the left leg under the knee. Bend the knee outward and lift the leg along the floor, then rest the bent leg. Your knee braces the left foot to keep the leg stable. Press on the buttock (2 breaths) and then along the back, going from lower left back upward and then down the right side of the back.

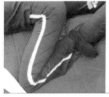 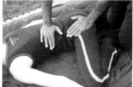 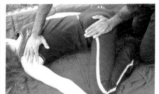 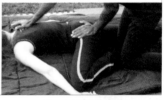

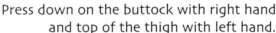

Press down on the buttock with right hand and top of the thigh with left hand.

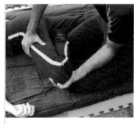

Straighten the leg and pull the leg. Bend the knee and press the foot. Lift the knee carefully and press the thigh.

With your hand under the knee, lift the leg as tolerated. Apply pressure by squeezing the thigh with the right hand.

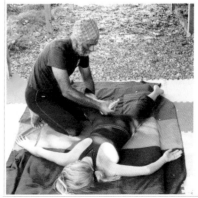 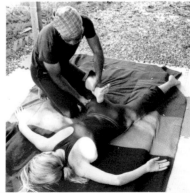

109

Gently straighten the leg and pull it back ,stretching the leg.
Pull legs back lifting them a few inches.
Apply pressure on the bottom of the foot with your fist or hands.
Press at several points.

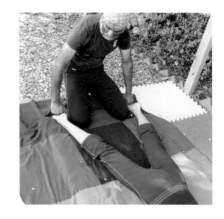

RECEIVER ON STOMACH: UPPER BODY
(don't press on the spine)

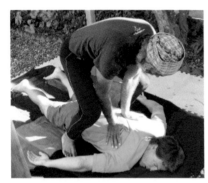

Press on the lower back with your hands.

Hold each pressure spot for two breaths.

Keep moving your hands a few inches until you have pressed all of the left and right side of the back.

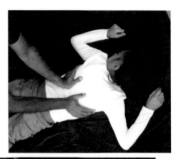

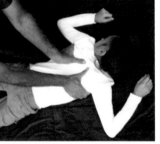

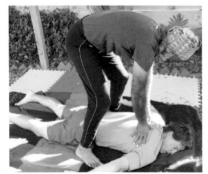

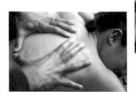

Press on the head gently and use the fingers to gently squeeze at several different points.

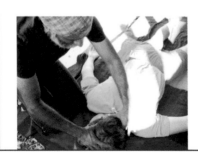

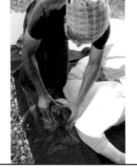

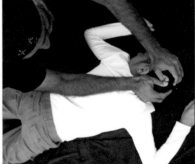

Vishram with Ropes

For a receiver who can handle more pressure, one can hold the ropes and use the full body weight for pressure. This should be done carefully, until the giver is confident that the receiver can handle the pressure. Never press on the knee, spine, neck or head. You can also keep one foot on the ground and use the other foot to gently shift your weight to slowly build pressure.

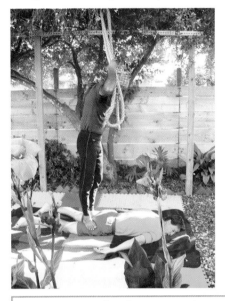
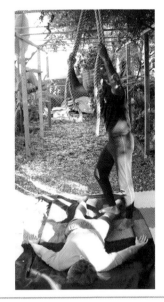
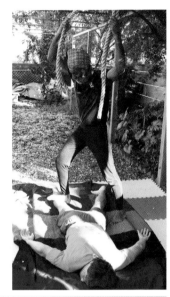

A very comforting stretch

The receiver sits comfortably with the torso erect (giver stands). Interlock the fingers with hands behind the neck.

Giver places his knee gently against the receiver's back, to the side of the spine.

Gently pull the elbows back. After stretching for 3-4 breaths, receiver lowers the hands and presses the neck and shoulder area.

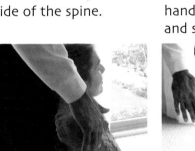
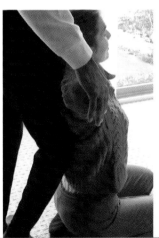
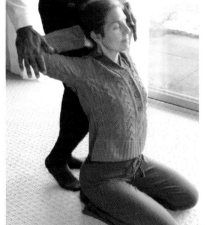

After the vishram yoga is completed, have the receiver lie under a blanket for warmth and comfort.

ਮਨ ਤੂੰ ਜੋਤ ਸਵਾਰੂਪ ਹੈ ਅਪਨਾ ਮੂਲ ਪਛਾਨ

Man toon jot swaroop hain apna mool pachhaan

Within you lies the light, recognize your worth.

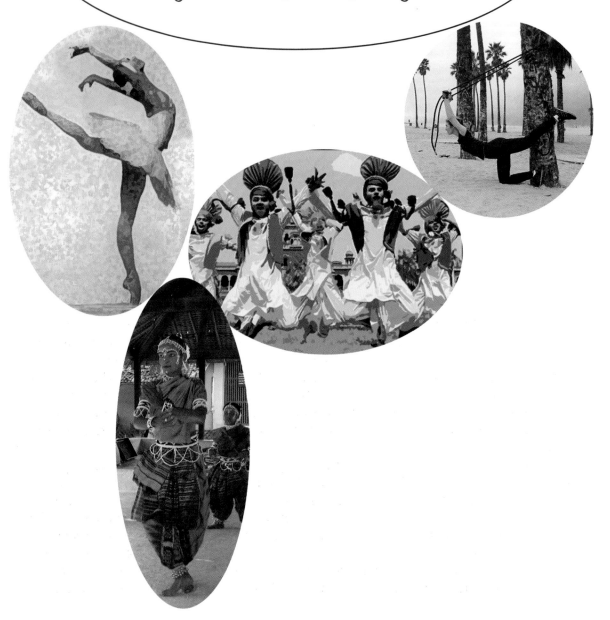

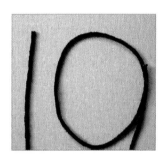

SELF-AWARENESS:
Inner Resonances and Allergies

Natural Way and Your Resonance

All of us want to be happy. We want to be healthy, optimistic, and we want our lives to be filled with joy. But, more often than not, for a variety of reasons, this goal is not attained. A key to happiness and optimism is self-awareness and awareness of the world in which we live. If we do not know ourselves, how do we know what gives us happiness? If we live in an environment that doesn't support our inner resonances we will feel stifled. But first we need to be aware—of ourselves and of the outside world.

We all have similar basic needs. We need food to nourish our bodies, shelter and clothes to protect it from the elements, companionship to nurture our social needs, and solitude to meditate on deeper questions. Beyond these basics lie a wide variety of individual wishes. Some of us enjoy watching movies, some relish reading a book, some like to enjoy fine spirits, some prefer to sit and meditate. All of these desires help create a diverse human experience and a lively economy. As our understanding of the human body is increasing we are finding that much of what gives us drive and pleasure is encoded into our DNA. Even our level of happiness under normal conditions appears to be linked to our DNA. As does our individual propensity to handle alcohol, risky behavior, overeating, etc. Our desires are also linked to our friends and to our society.

Consider a concert pianist who is planning to play for a big event. A great deal of time is spent on tuning the piano and making sure the instruments' "resonances" are as perfect as possible. But if the concert is played in a hall with poor acoustics and outside noise, the best recital will become frustrating. The hall, its design, etc., provides what we'll call the "Natural Way" of the outside world. The integration and coupling of the "inner resonances" with the "Natural Way" is essential for harmony.

Yoga practice in general and RussaYog practice in particular places the mind and body in a state (calm-alert) where one can answer the following questions:

What are my inherent resonances?

Does the local Natural Way support my resonances?

Can I alter my inner resonances or develop new ones?

INHERENT RESONANCE

You need not be a musician to realize that each sound of a musical instrument is unique. You may alter the sounds to create a range of sound frequencies, but a drum is unlikely to sound like a horn. A guitar is unlikely to sound like a piano. Knowing the inherent resonances of musical instruments and learning how to manipulate the keys, strings, pressure points, etc., allows our energy to be channeled into beautiful music.

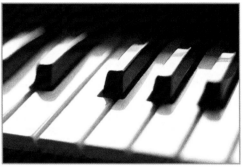

Say you do an activity then find out on some scale how much pleasure or satisfaction you received from it. Some activities give you no pleasure or may even cause you to be depressed. But some give you a very high return of pleasure. As in musical instruments those are your resonances. The term resonance is used in music or electronics and one does a simple

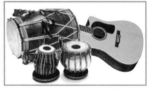

experiment to find the resonance of a musical instrument or an electronic circuit. A small signal (whose properties, like frequency, can be varied) is inputted into the instrument or the circuit, and the output is measured. The input could come from a tuning fork or an electronic oscillator that can generate a wide range of frequencies. If the output is high the circuit has a resonance for the particular input. In the process of the experiment there should be no distraction, otherwise the conclusions will be corrupted. A string instrument has certain resonances that can be controlled by the length and tension of the string. Your radio or television uses a circuit that has a resonance that can be adjusted to that of a particular channel. We can also learn to tune our resonance so we can derive pleasure from many different sources.

If you have a guitar you can pluck the strings and create a range of notes. However, the guitar does not have the same resonances as a drum. No matter how hard a guitar virtuoso plucks the strings, he cannot make the guitar sound like a drum. Unless he considers that guitar does not only have strings. It has a body, too. You may have heard of innovative players use the guitar body to create sounds unlike the strings. By broadening the dimension of the instrument new resonances can be created.

Finding our inherent resonance is a critical part of happiness and wealth building. If you do not know your inner resonance you may end up using a trumpet to create the sounds of a violin. In most cultures a self-aware person is considered wise. The better you know yourself—in all aspects—the better you will be at fulfilling your desires. For example, on a very mundane level, many of us have some allergies to foods. Allergies are like the inverse of resonances (we will use the term anti-resonances for them). Does it not make sense to avoid foods that you know are allergenic to you? On a social and spiritual level we can determine what our resonances are and what our anti-resonances are. We can employ a variation of the technique used by engineers for electronic circuits. This technique may be called meditation-participation technique. You calm yourself by meditating so there are minimal distractions. Then participate in an activity, and again calmly reflect to figure out if you got the pleasure you wanted. It is important to note that our inherent resonances will change as we get older or wiser.

Knowledge of our inherent resonances allows us to do things that we enjoy. You channel your wealth into these activities. If you know you enjoy dancing you can spend your money taking a dance class, instead of going to see a tractor-pull contest. Also, if you know your resonances you can arrange to go into professions that allow you to have fun while your accumulate wealth.

To learn about your own resonances, do the following exercise.

Assemble a list of 5 items in your inner resonances from the following categories:

PHYSICAL	BODY EXPERIENCES	MENTAL	SOCIAL	SPIRITUAL	CHALLENGES
Touch	Squeeze	Problem-solving	Conversation	Feeling/giving love	Poor health
Smell	Stretch	Memorization	Food sharing	Infinitesimal	Poverty
Taste	Movement	Language skills	Dancing	and Infinite	Unhappy
Sight	Play	Writing	People-		family life
Hearing	Balance	Music	watching		Social/
Sex	Painting	Shopping			cultural bindings
		Fantasy			
		On-line gaming			

Once you have a list of inherent resonances you should identify the cost to indulge these resonances. Some resonances cost more wealth, while others may be free. If you want to be in 70 degrees F temperature in Las Vegas in July be prepared to pay for the electricity. But in San Diego you may do so for no cost. By being in touch with your resonances and being aware of their cost, you can make wise decisions about indulging your pleasures based on the wealth you have.

LOCAL NATURAL WAY

We know from Physics that the laws of Nature are independent of time and space. The laws that control aerodynamics of an airplane are the same in Chicago and Tokyo. However, the same laws of Nature can produce differences in the Natural Way at different places. There are differences in weather patterns, and oceans, rivers, and rainfalls are geographically different. Public policies, social customs, religions, and economies are different, leading to variations in local Natural Ways. These differences manifest themselves in different ways. In San Francisco you will have no need of air conditioning, while in Phoenix you can physically get hurt without it. A doctor in Bangladesh may be lucky to earn $5000 per year, while a doctor in USA can pull down half a million dollars. The economic models in developed countries allow for ease in generation of wealth and in use of wealth to create diverse experiences. This is not to say that in poorer countries it's always more difficult to live in the Natural Way. In many poorer countries the Natural Way allows for close friendships and kinships. In economically powerful countries people have to often travel thousands of miles to see their parents or grandparents for a few days out of a year. The high mobility necessary for professional development allows little time to nurture friendships. The important issue is not which Natural Way is better, but which one meshes best with your inherent resonances. Even if you are unable, for various reasons, to live in an area where the Natural Way is best for you, at least you will know what is the price to be paid.

To check on how well your local Natural Way blends with your inherent resonances ask the following question: How much wealth or energy is needed to be able to create an awesome activity that provides you pleasure? In some cases the answer is simple: we can look up an airfare for a trip to Hawaii; we can find the cost of that sharp convertible; we can figure out the cost of air conditioning, etc. However, it is often difficult to figure out what the cost of an experience is. What is the cost of a hug from your son or daughter? What is the cost of a happy home?

Diversifying our Inner Resonances

Our personalities are diverse enough that we have more than one inherent resonance. We like a variety of foods, we like a variety of music. We like a variety of sports, films, and video games. We like different subjects in school. Moreover, most of us may not have experienced enough activities to know all of the different experiences that resonate with our being. To know and develop as many of our resonances as possible is important for the following reasons:

VERY EXPENSIVE DOMINANT RESONANCE

The activity we enjoy may be very expensive and may take up all of our wealth. For example, if you enjoy skiing, but you have to travel a thousand miles to find a ski resort, you will be either spending a lot of money satisfying your desire, or you may feel deprived. If you find out that there are other sports that give you equal pleasure, but don't cost so much, you will greatly increase your happiness.

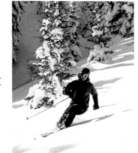

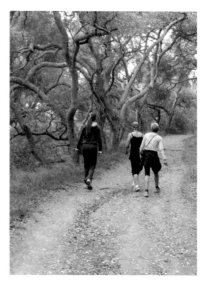

HIGHLY ADDICTIVE DOMINANT RESONANCE

What if you have a genetic makeup that gives you a propensity to become an addict to certain activities. What if you enjoy a highly addictive resonance like smoking or gambling or drinking? These activities may give you great pleasure, but they may then take you down a path where you are unable to function as your true self. If you have a broad range of resonances, you could find one that takes less of a toll on your life, but gives you the pleasure you seek.

A DOMINANT RESONANCE THAT IS ILLEGAL

We live in societies that are bound by laws. Sometimes these laws may not seem fair, but one has to abide by them (or work to change them) or face the wrath of the legal system. Resonances linked to illegal drugs trap a lot of people. As is generally true of most resonances, it takes a certain threshold of participation before a resonance becomes hard-wired to your body. Once established, a resonance is very difficult to reverse. You are better off developing and finding resonances that are healthy for you.

Changing Our Resonances

Can we change our inherent resonances? When a musician plays a guitar he can alter the note by adjusting the length of the string. However, a guitar cannot sound like a trumpet. A trumpet cannot produce a drum sound. Increasingly, social and medical scientists are finding that people have some inherent resonances that are genetic in nature. These resonances are so dominant that they cannot influence them merely through strong will power. However, even the strongest resonances can be modified and controlled through some basic principles:

1. Couple with others: A social group can modify an individual's behavior in both positive and negative ways. Just as a group of musicians can jam and create experiences that none of the players can do individually, in groups we can elicit qualities and vices that we didn't know existed. This is one reason why good friends are so precious. Some people can do fun things in a crowd of strangers that they cannot do on their own. People can dance wildly in clubs and crowds. Even with a pet, one can enjoy experiences that one may not enjoy by oneself.

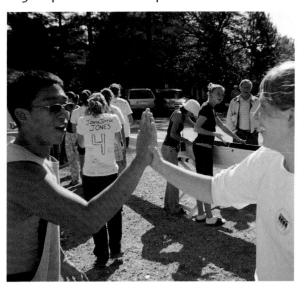

2. Selectively feed resonances: If you want certain resonances to be suppressed you can ensure that they receive no energy and time from you. On the other hand, ensure that there is a lot of nourishment for resonances you want nurtured. In other words, prioritize your life. If alcohol creates a

dominant resonance in your life, ensure that you don't have alcohol around. Instead, nurture a different resonance, say, exercising or going out with sober friends. Most of us are not aware of all of our resonances because, for various reasons, we have not nourished them.

3. Grow new resonances: Yes, you can develop new resonances through travel, education, art,...Just as increasing the length of a string on an instrument gives it a wider range, your growth can open new resonances.

It may well be that your genetics determine your resonances, but that is no reason to give up the endeavor to make your life more multi-dimensional. The short paragraphs we have noted here are described in long articles and books on nature-versus-nurture debates. Books are available in any bookstore on addictions ranging from food-related issues to alcohol and cocaine and how to overcome them. By no means is the short description here suggestive that it is easy to develop new resonances or nullify resonances that have become dominant in our lives. But it is important to note that it is possible to do so.

4. Let yourself have pleasure: When a child goes to Disneyland everything is so exciting. Scores of experiences packaged in the form of rides—joyful, scary, thrilling, dizzying; shows—dancers, pirates, Mickey Mouse; fantasy creations—castles, ships, forts—give the child (and the child in adults) a wonderful day. The Universe is a much bigger collection of fun-filled experiences. However, just like at Disneyland, in the Universe we need to let ourselves have fun. If a child gets tangled up in a bush in Disneyland he will miss the fun. If we are tangled up in ignorance, worries, anxieties, pessimism, we will also miss the fun.

RussaYog is centered around chardi kala and anand—optimism and joy. One may say these words represent the belief system of RussaYog and everything is designed to create this experience.

For some people joyful living may mean reclusive living. For some it may mean ascetic living. If these choices are made freely, then that is the right path for them. And, hopefully, these choices have not left behind people (especially children) who were counting on them. Having been born in India and spending decades travelling there, my experience is that too many times the "sadhus" and "yogis" have left behind pits of unfulfilled promises to their families. However, undoubtedly there are genuinely "free" spirits as well who have earned their freedom by fulfilling obligations, not by dumping them.

For those who are not recluses or who do not want to lead an ascetic life, how do we balance the pleasures and hardships of what life brings? Life brings pleasures of the senses, to the mind, during social activities, and pleasures of the spiritual realm. Life also offers the challenges of disease, poverty, betrayal, hatred, and family burdens. Since yoga is all about coherence and RussaYog folds in the element of joyful balance, it makes sense that, as far as possible, we should use what life offers and design a feast for ourselves. A finely prepared feast includes ingredients that, as a whole, are delicious and healthful. But if only one ingredient is consumed exclusively, illness is not far behind.

In the RussaYog session a yogi learns to balance the hold on the rope. The placement of the foot or knee, the adjustment of forces... create a joyful experience. In life also the pleasures and challenges (responsibilities) can be balanced to create a sensual life. By sensual we do not just mean physical sensuality alone (an important component), but we mean pleasures involving all of our senses.

Let us summarize the concepts covered in this chapter:

• Develop self-awareness to understand what provides you pleasure.
Also identify your source of allergies.
• Continuously strive to expand the range of activities that provide you joy.
• Decrease the threshold point where your pleasure kicks in—
work to eliminate the friction of worry, anxiety, and prejudice.
This will allow you to experience pleasure with minimal effort and waste.
• Beware to not let pleasureful activities become addictive.
• Have a mutli-dimensional life.
• It is hard to have a joyful life without optimism and it is hard to be optimistic if we have a me-vs-them attitude.

It is up to each individual to find a balanced life. It is useful to develop a chart of menus/recipes just like a good chef does to whip up a fun dish, even when the perfect ingredients are not available. (See the table on page 115.)

Also identify forces that diminish your chances of achieving joyful states. Make efforts to reduce these damping factors. If needed, you may have to avoid people who pull you down—just like you avoid foods that are unhealthy for you.

Most importantly, give yourself permission to have fun and enjoy life. And use RussaYog to strengthen yourself, so you participate in life and enjoy it.

अपन flexibility यश strength मान poise

Your karmic wealth determines
how far you are from enlightenment
ਕਰਮੀ ਆਪੋ ਆਪਨੀ ਕੇ ਨੇੜੇ ਕੇ ਦੂਰ
Karmi apo aapni ke nerai ke dur

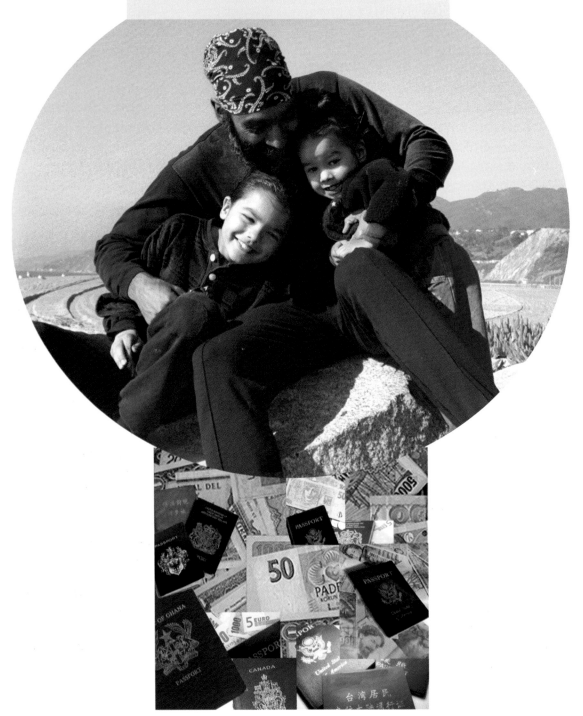

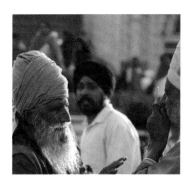

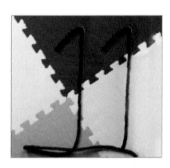

KARMIC WEALTH AND LAWS OF KARMA

A common theme that runs through all Indian philosophies and religions is that of "karma" and "karmic wealth." Just as Western-style capitalism is based on material wealth, Indian philosophies are based on karmic wealth which is a larger view of our total wealth. Different Indian faiths may have different interpretations of karmic wealth, but the general concepts are pervasive. In fact, one may argue that belief in karma is what allows the incredibly diverse population (languages, racial make-up, religions, etc.) of India to call themselves Indian.

For anyone using the concepts of yoga and RussaYog described here it is important to examine the notions of karmic wealth and the general laws of karma. If you go to any major bookstore you will find dozens of books on financial planning, wealth growth, early retirement, etc. We are intrigued by wealthy people. Sometimes we envy them, sometimes we try to emulate them, sometimes we wait to see if something bad happens to them. Rarely do we ignore them. Most of us want to be wealthy. Wealth seems to be almost equivalent to being free. And our daily experience usually does confirm this attitude. If we have some extra money it gives us the freedom to do whatever we want.

Karmic Wealth

Some life experiences are fun, while others are painful. In some events we participate voluntarily, in others we are forced to participate. Sometimes we want certain experiences, but are unable to achieve them. In an ice-storm we want to be on a sunny beach. Sick, lying in bed, we want to feel light and healthy. There are many tools that allow us to create desired experiences for ourselves, but none are as universal and powerful as wealth. You've won a million dollars! These words create a sense of relief, freedom, new experiences, growth! Dollars, real estate, stocks, bonds...that's what wealth is associated with. In reality, wealth is much more encompassing than this.

The most important purpose of wealth is to allow us to convert one life experience to another. We need wealth because we may not be satisfied with our situation. Of course, the more one accepts one's situation the lesser the need for wealth. Wealth is like the gasoline we put in our cars. Without gasoline ours cars are stuck. With a full tank we can have the freedom of traveling, seeing new sights, and literally changing our station in life. Unfortunately, we have a healthier relation with gasoline than we do with wealth. Few people worry about gasoline (except in cases of a oil-embargo or a major storm like Katrina in New Orleans, which wipes out gas stations). We think about where we will go in our car, what we will do, the fun we will have, or the work we will do. We are focused on the experience that gasoline will provide us—not the gasoline itself. Our relation to wealth should be similar. The enjoyment of a life experience is more important than wealth. Wealth is a tool. Once we realize wealth is a tool, we may expand the definition of wealth to any tool that allows us to create desired experiences. It makes sense to choose the wealth which is most efficient in providing the desired life experience. For example, to obtain some life experiences you may want to cash in your dollars. For others you may want to make a phone call to a well-connected uncle. Certain life experiences can only be provided by a friend, a lover, a son or daughter, or a parent. The term karmic wealth represents any kind of wealth that allows us to create karma (action, experience). Material wealth is but one of the many forms of karmic wealth, yet is currently one the most discernible forms of wealth in modern life.

1. VALUED WEALTH

This is wealth that is well recognized by the markets— dollars, real estate, gold, stocks, bonds, etc. Use of this wealth to obtain experiences is simple and well understood. You can go to a store and buy an ice-cream cone. You can buy an airline ticket and travel to Brazil. You can buy a powerful car and go for a drive. Valued wealth allows you to buy almost everything in life and is definitely the most versatile form of wealth. It is like electricity (comparing wealth and energy). With electricity you can light a bulb, cool your fridge, listen to music, see a television program, heat a cup of water, etc. There are some exceptions to what you can do with electricity. Usually you cannot ride your car to work using electricity. For that you need gasoline.

2. RELATIONSHIP WEALTH

Relationship wealth is usually not recognized by the market. This wealth may be as important as valued wealth and may include friendships, family ties, marriage, etc. You can use this wealth, but the rules of exchange are fuzzy and you may not always know them. Your aunt may one day take you to Paris. Your uncle may buy you a nice suit and take you to a fancy restaurant. You may even fail college and yet get a high paying job in your father's friend's business. Normally we take the unvalued wealth for granted, since it is in the background. But if we lose our friends, our parents, or our children, we realize how valuable the relations were. In comparing wealth to energy, unvalued wealth is like sunshine. It makes us feel good and we are uplifted by it. We can't place a clear value on it, but without sunshine we get depressed and disheartened.

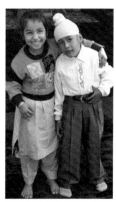

3. CATALYTIC WEALTH

There is a special kind of wealth that allows you to lower barriers and open doors in your pursuit of certain experiences. Catalytic wealth is not used up, as is the case for other kinds of wealth. When you buy a brand new car you have to give up $30,000 (or more, dependng upon the car). But with catalytic wealth the car dealer may just let you have the car because you are a celebrity (a movie star) or you belong to a certain select club and can introduce him to the exclusive clientele. There are a number of types of catalytic wealth that lower barriers for the possessor. Often we are not willing to acknowledge or are not proud that barriers have been lowered for us. But catalytic wealth is used all the time. Important types of catalytic wealth include charisma and optimism. Other examples of catalytic wealth are caste, race, skin color, memberships in exclusive clubs, exceptional beauty, and national origin.

4. SACRED WEALTH

This is wealth that you are not willing to part with because of faith, cultural values, or social taboos. For example, if someone offers you a million dollars (or a fun-filled life experience) in exchange for your son or daughter, you would reject it without a thought. Similarly, in most societies young women will not exchange sex for money. A person with high integrity will not lie to achieve material wealth. In some families there are heirlooms that are outside the market forces. In other societies the rivers and trees are sacred and should not be exploited. As societies

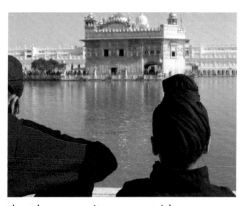

change sometimes sacred wealth is cashed in and when that happens it can provide a huge jump in valued wealth. Often this happens in immigrant communities where certain taboos or beliefs are broken as a result of the new life, resulting in many positive and some negative experiences.

While driving your car on a curvy mountain road you notice guard rails along the road, particularly where the road is narrow and a small miscalculation can send you tumbling into a crevice. Sacred wealth is like a guard rail of life. It does not seem important until a mishap occurs. By cashing in this guard rail one can instantly gain valued wealth. But one has to be careful in this exchange. Of course, some guard rails are placed in areas where the road is wide and flat and are not needed. Or some may fall down and create roadblocks. It certainly makes sense to get rid of them. Some sacred wealth may involve beliefs or rituals that tax your intelligence or degrade other humans. It may not make sense to hold on to them.

Sacred wealth is like nuclear energy. It is hidden away and one doesn't notice it. However, it is enormous if converted. And after conversion everything transforms. In the sun nuclear energy is released as hydrogen atoms converted to helium atoms. In a nuclear reactor uranium transforms, leaving behind nuclear waste.

Capitalism and Karmic Wealth

While dealing with these four categories of wealth we should recognize that free markets only understand valued wealth and, therefore, only give us feedback on our valued wealth. In a marketplace when people interact with us they pay attention to our valued wealth. Unless we are in the company of wise men and women, it is natural for most of us to lose perspective of our unvalued wealth. Gradually, as we make decisions about life choices, we learn to only consider our valued wealth.

In a culture where logic and rational thought is dominant whenever a clash between valued wealth and unvalued wealth occurs, valued wealth usually comes out on top. Thus, in a market economy, with few exceptions, a friendship always loses out to a promotion and a move to a distant city. Most modern economies rely on this principle. Companies know they can transfer employees with a promise of a raise and promotion. This is not a moral lapse—it is a natural intelligent choice between something that is clearly spelled out (a job contract) and one that is kind of fuzzy.

In Chapter 2 (see page 14) we discussed the four stages of karma-fruit relationship. We discussed the stages of saturation and catastrophic failure. Yes, we need a certain minimum material wealth, otherwise our lives can become miserable. But one should be able to find higher purposes in life than simply accumulating more wealth. While the term obesity is used for people who are very heavy in body, it can also be applied to people who have excessive baggage of material wealth. After all, money is given to us in exchange for our lives. It is important to develop other ingredients of karmic wealth—relational and especially, sacred wealth.

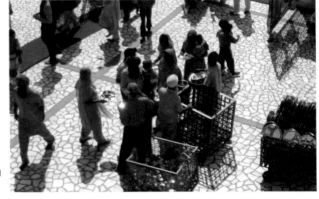

One has to acknowledge that market forces and capitalism have had a positive impact on basic human living conditions, perhaps more so than religions and wars. Markets have succeeded in making changes for the good, where wars and religion have failed. The impact can be seen in race relations, gender relations, and freedom to travel and pursue individual talents. Many race and gender barriers have fallen because the capital markets demanded they be brought down.

The purpose of this chapter is to allow you to make an informed decision when you consider your valued wealth and your unvalued or sacred wealth. The informed consumer is one of the pillars of a free market. Tomes on financial planning have been pretty good in providing consumers information on how to price stocks, bonds etc., and how to build valued wealth. But they don't deal with unvalued wealth.

Trading-in Life Experiences: Laws of Karma

The basic laws of karma are not so different from the accounting laws that allow you to earn money at a job, deposit or invest the money, and then use it to go shopping. Of course, with karmic laws you are dealing with your entire karmic wealth, not just money. But who is the Banker? Who sets the laws? Who enforces the laws? Every country has its version of a central bank, rules and regulations, and law enforcement agencies. In the greater karmic domain Nature (Creator, God, the Great Spirit...) runs the machinery of banking. Men and women intervene to take charge of karmic laws and try to enforce their own versions by force or philosophical persuasion. But let us first take a general view of the karmic laws.

We carry out efforts in our lives and accumulate karma. Good karma, bad karma, neutral karma. Life is just an exchange of one life effort or experience for another. The effort is kirit which, according to karmic laws, earns us karma. The karma can then be cashed in to obtain joy/sorrow. Religions have come up with kirits that provide, according to them, the best way to accumulate karma. Charity, love, rituals, pilgrimages, feeding the Brahmins, marrying within the caste, etc., are some of the ways we can accumulate good karma. Drinking, drugs, murder, too much fun, etc., are ways we accumulate bad karma. Of course, not all of these man-made laws make sense.

God or Creator's laws are supposed to ensure a fair and reliable system which keeps track of each persons' karma and allows us to cash it in. When we cash in the karma, we are enjoying the fruits of labor. This is ਭੋਗ bhog. The threefold effort-laws of exchange-enjoyment or ਕਿਰਤ–ਹੁਕਮ–ਭੋਗ kirit-hukam-bhog then form our lifecycle.

Effort	Laws of Karma	Fruit
ਕਿਰਤ	ਹੁਕਮ	ਭੋਗ

Some aspects of karma seem to be set by Nature and laws of nature. If you follow well-known laws of nutrition, hygiene, and health you can see a direct connection between your action and the positive karma you accumulate. In addition, each society has somehow decided what constitutes good and bad karma. Karma can take the form of birth into a high caste, birth as a man, birth into a specific race, etc. Birth as a woman, a person with dark skin, or the wrong passport, are areas where negative karma is assigned at birth with no obvious connection to any natural law. Reform movements around the world have tried to redefine the definitions of good karma.

Unfortunately, the exchange of considerable amount of karma is usually not governed by any Natural laws, but by man-made laws. In many ways the laws of market-based karma are the most democratic and unbiased set of karmic laws. Compare, for example, the accounting laws for money with the laws of caste system traditionally followed in India (discrimination based upon caste is illegal in India today). In India the caste karma has created tremendous pains for the lowest class or Shudras. Elaborate myths have been developed to give the Brahmin-born family special "exchange rates." In Western countries the white race has been assumed to possess special karma just by being born into a white family. Once again special "exchange rates" are reserved for this class. And in almost all societies a man has been given extra privileges over a woman. It is hard not to admire the benefits of the market forces in leveling out these special exchange rates.

A passport remains one of the easiest ways to accumulate karma. A person born in USA has a starting karma much larger than a person born in Bangladesh or Liberia. Just by moving to USA such a person can instantly increase his or her wealth. Millions of immigrants know this! The ability to convert effort into wealth is much more efficient in the USA than in less developed economies. In fact, every group in power has tried to develop a set of karmic laws favorable to itself.

LAWS OF KARMA

The laws of karma are very much like the rules of accounting. Some accounting rules seem rooted in universal values. Others seem quite arbitrary. However, once the rules are established the outcome is not very difficult to follow (provided there is no cheating). Karma and its use is just a high level of accounting. It involves detailed mathematics. Most of the time we can see the laws of karma at work. If we exercise, we become healthier. If we help another human being we not only feel good, we are also helped by others. We do see the cause and effect that a simple karmic law implies. However, often unexpected things occur which seemingly have no connection to what we may have done. Most so-called miracles are an attempt to explain these events.

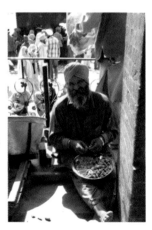

Consider the following events that seem to defy any law of accounting.
• You exercise, eat properly, and rest but you get cancer.
• You work hard and do your job responsibly, but you get fired.
• You go out of your way to help a stranded motorist and he robs you.
• You save money all your life and build a beautiful home. A storm destroys it.
• You goof off in school, party all day, and then win a million dollars in a lottery.
What we find in life is that many events are easily explained, but many (and often the more important ones) seem to just happen out of the blue. So what are the laws of karma? To understand the laws we make a comparison with the laws of accounting by examining various forms of accounts. You can go to a bank and set up any number of accounts. Let us see what happens when you make a deposit and make a withdrawal:

• Individual Account: If you have an individual account where you are the only one allowed to make a deposit and withdrawal the rules are very simple. When you have some money you can place it in the bank. If the bank is an international bank you can make deposits in dollars, pounds, euros, yen, etc. The bank knows the exchange rates and credits your account. If you make a withdrawal your account value decreases. The bank is generous and sometimes lets your balance become negative, trusting you to make up the deficit. Every month, or anytime you can check your account. A good bank never makes an error. The individual account operates in a manner that is easy to understand and is predictable.

• Joint Account: You go to a bank and open a joint account with your spouse or a friend or a business partner. The joint account also has clear rules, but they treat you and your partner as one entity. Therefore while dealing with the joint account if you fail to take the "two-is-one" approach, you will be surprised. You may one day examine the account expecting to find a balance of $10,000, but instead you find $15,000! You discover from the bank that your partner had made a deposit a few hours prior. Another day you check the account and find just a few hundred dollars remain. You rush to the bank and discover that your partner just withdrew most of the money. Eventually you may realize that the joint account is useful, but you can no longer think of the cause-effect relation with only you in the picture. You must broaden your sense of self. Once you do that the rules become clear and make sense.

• Corporate Account: You go one step further and get involved in a business with a dozen other partners. Now you go to the bank and set up a corporate account. The bank describes the rules of the account to all of you. Anyone can make a deposit or withdrawal. Now the bank statements become even more unexpected. You see wild fluctuations which obviously arise because so many people are involved. Now you have to expand your sense of self even further. If you can do that, the account becomes understandable.

• A Global Mutual Fund Account: You find out about another type of account which allows you to invest in mutual funds across the world which allows you to earn profit from the stock market, yet make withdrawals anytime you wish. Once again the rules are simple: you make a deposit and inform the bank how you want your money distributed. Now the unpredictability of your account magnifies– even though the rules appear simple. The stock market is so complex that your fund becomes unrelated to what you, individually, are doing. The economy performs well and your value increases. The market collapses and your value plummets. Now you have to expand your sense of self to include all of the corporations that comprise your investments.

Only if you are isolated from others can you apply a simplistic law of karma—a good karma can be cashed in by me and there is a direct link between what I sow and what I reap. In more complex situations you can only understand and, therefore, use the laws of karma by expanding your sense of self. For example, if you contract a disease unrelated to your diet and exercise habits, it may be related to the bad karma of pollutants in the city you live or the bad karma of the food industry upon which you depend. Sometimes we have choices about which relationships we are involved in, but sometimes we have little choice. Of course, the answer is not to isolate oneself from the world. There are obvious benefits to couple with others. When you couple with others you must realize that if you do good things, others may benefit from your action. Conversely, you may benefit from others' good deeds. Also, if someone else does something bad, you will suffer. It would be silly to apply the laws of an individual account to a corporate account.

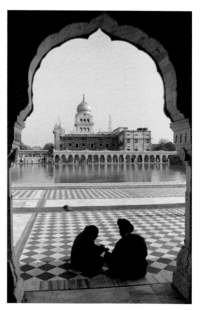

WHAT IF THE KARMIC LAWS ARE BIASED?

Suppose you open one of the accounts described and one of the following occurs:

1) Prejudice: The bank (or brokerage) contract states, in fine print, that for people born in May (which happens to be your birth month) a fee of an extra 10% of your balance will be deducted every year. On the other hand, if you are born in December you will receive a 10% bonus from the bank. In this case, the laws of the account are stacked against you or for you for no logical reason. The caste system and the race system is an example of such a deviant karmic system. In most societies the laws of karma are biased, and are not based on completely equal treatment of people.

2) Theft: You find that the bank managers are skimming from your account balance. They are stealing from you. You work hard and a colleague takes credit for your work and gets a raise, but you do not. This kind of violation is harder to take than the biased laws about which you are pre-informed. At least if you are aware of the bias in advance you can prepare for it—and eventually fight it.

The important point in understanding the laws of karma is that they are complex and, although for many cases a clear path can be delineated from the effort to the reward, in some cases it is hard to describe this path. Social reformers have continually fought against the biases in karmic laws set up by men and women. The civil rights movement in United States was an effort to balance the laws. Criminal laws make an effort to deter theft in our lives.

IS THERE A BIAS IN NATURAL LAWS?

The creation of biased laws are motivated by self-preservation or a "my-group-first" mindset. But is Nature biased? Children are born with different mental and physical abilities. They are born into rich families and poor families. They are born in countries with differing resources. So how are all people created equally?

Clearly Nature ensures that what is created is unique. People are not born with identical assets. One can only argue that in the path that really matters, we have an equal chance. We all have a chance to make our life joyful. Empirically it seems true that a billionaire can be unhappy (or happy) just as a poor poet can be happy (or unhappy). All of us can enlighten ourselves to reach happiness. Fortunately, sustained happiness depends more on enlightenment than on wealth and possessions. In that sense Nature has given us all equal opportunity. If we regard ourselves as finite beings there will always be a comparison with others, resulting in feeling lesser or greater than others. However, if we feel connected to the infinite, comparisons disappear.

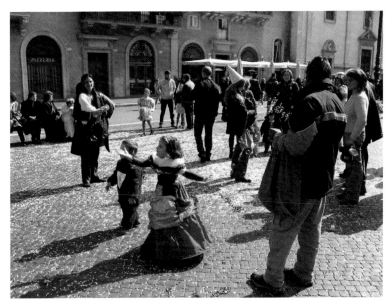

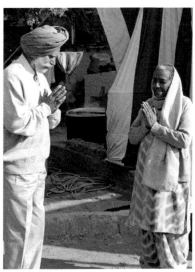

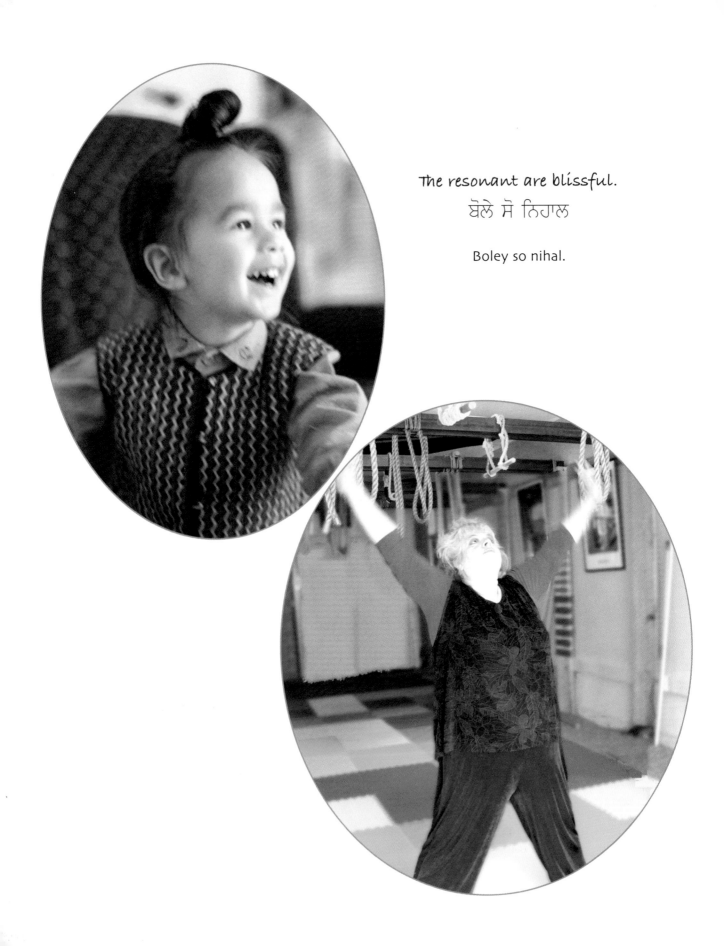

The resonant are blissful.

ਬੋਲੇ ਸੋ ਨਿਹਾਲ

Boley so nihal.

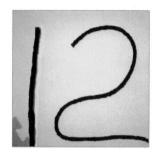

YOGA AND WELLNESS

This book is primarily written for people in the developed world where starvation and deprivation is becoming extinct. With the United States at the helm, obesity rates in these countries are rapidly increasing. Lack of a balanced diet, lack of exercise, high-stress jobs, a car-based lifestyle, etc., have made health care a very big business. A large fraction of health care concerns fixing problems that may not have arisen if lifestyle changes were made, like incorporating an hour of exercise a day, and consuming a fiber, fruit, lentils and vegetable-based diet. One does not have to be extremely strict—the human body can handle some poor food choices. Moderate consumption of desserts, alcohol, and meats will not make you sick.

The human body is a wonderfully-designed machine that can self heal and stay healthy—if treated properly. A RussaYog-based lifestyle involving pranayam, bal-lila, and veer-lila, along with embracing the spirit of chardi kala is an excellent way to live the modern life. Pranayam and asans have been shown to help in reducing blood pressure and heart disease. Also, a calm-alert mind doesn't resort to high-fat foods and poor rest-sleep habits when confronted with stress.

Western style empirical-based health care and yoga-based personal health care are the best antidote to the stresses of modern life. The body and the environment are so complex that we need more empirical studies of how yoga benefits illnesses. If one listens to every "new-age" health specialist (including those promoting yoga, mega-vitamins, herbal remedies, and special diets) one can expect that every disease can be cured with simple concoctions. This, of course, is not true. How does one sort out the genuine claims from made-up claims?

Science and Self-Awareness:
Well-Being in a Complex Environment

How does one find truth in a complex system? You are very sick, nursing a fever of 104 degrees F. Your aunt comes by and repeats a mantra that a sadhu has given her and puts a smudge of ash on your forehead. Next morning you feel great. Should you start depending upon the sadhu to cure all of your medical ailments? Or was your body already in the process of overpowering the disease when your aunt showed up? The health field is a complex system. Hundreds of forces are at play and the outcome is subtly dependent upon their interplay. Someone drinks tulsi tea for three weeks and his ulcers are gone. Someone did a headstand and his migraines disappeared. How do we know what is real and what is a fluke?

Science has developed the field of statistics and probability in order to understand complex systems. Statistics explain the concept of what will happen on average, and what is the probability of a deviation from the average to occur. You flip a coin 10 times. The most probable outcome is that you will get 5 heads and 5 tails. But there is a one in 1,024 chance that you will get all 10 heads or all 10 tails. It can happen that your cousin, Bill Luckyflip, tosses the coin 10 times and gets heads 10 times. Should we attribute this to the fact that he meditates every morning? Clearly not. However, there is a desire to assign such unusual and unexpected events to some unrelated behavior. In Figure A we show the average number of times we will get various head and tail combinations if we flip a coin 10 times. To understand the benefits of yoga, meditation, and other practices, it is important to keep probabilities in mind.

Increasingly, students and teachers of yoga are appreciating that if yoga-based wellness is to become accepted as a respectable practice we must employ empirical techniques which are extension of what has been developed by science.

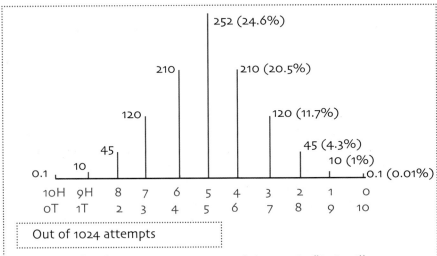

In 10 coin flips how many times (out of 1,024 coin flips) will we get various Head (H)/Tail (T) combinations? The most probable (a little over 25%) outcome is 5H and 5T. However, there is a one-in-a-thousand chance that you will get all 10 heads or all 10 tails. These fluke outcomes must not be attributed to anything but "luck."

Figure A

These techniques are, in fact, consistent with the principles of yoga. These techniques involve the three-fold process to determine the benefit of certain practices. These are: In a non-empirical approach, an outcome with miniscule probability may be declared as

1) carry out an experiment on the practice for a specified period of time, if possible, in a large cross-section of people;

2) interpret the results after setting your ego and preconceptions aside; and

3) use your own and others' intelligence to develop a theory of the benefits of the practice. Such a theory will place the outcome in terms of probabilities, not absolutes (as discussed for the case of flipped coins).

the outcome with certain probability. Recall the example of your lucky cousin who says with confidence, "Because I do yoga, every time I flip 10 coins, I will get 10 heads!"

Empirical techniques are being applied to yoga and more such work is needed. There is tremendous potential in alternative wellness approaches that include pranayam, asans, meditation, ayurvedic medicine, acupuncture, etc. However, if no empirical basis for the remedies exists, it opens doors to charlatans and fake claims. These, in turn, hurt legitimate wellness treatments. Keep in mind that statistics reflect an average. You can, through good practice, skew your own healing.

PREVENTION AS THE BEST MEDICINE

When you purchase a car a manual is included which tells you the maintenance schedule, for example, of the oil change, belt change, and radiator fluid change. If these maintenance guideline are followed, most cars can easily last for 15 years with no serious problems. If one ignores these guidelines, the car will get into serious problems. Granted, the human body is much more complex, however, certain similarities can be used for comparison. Whereas Western medicine has developed wonderful treatments and drugs, the business model often depends upon continual sickness. A self-aware person will avoid and prevent most health problems. Consider physical prevention issues: good nutrition habits, good rest habits, and a clean environment. For humans, emotional well-being is also critical. The ability to deal with situations that create anger, disappointment, and betrayal is very important, since simmering feelings of despair can result from life's stresses. Inability to deal with negative stress can also trigger additional biological pathways which can lead to physical illnesses, such as cancer, as well as psychological disorders. A RussaYog-based lifestyle can lead to:

• A strong, muscular body with a good sense of balance.

• An emotionally balanced mind. This is a mind that does not get caught up in blame or victimization syndrome (why me?), quick to get angry and frustrated.

These abilities, in turn, help prevent many health-related problems.

> "The chances of being healthy in old age are better than even for people who at mid-life have normal blood pressure, good grip strength, and several other physical characterisitics associated with being fit and active."
>
> "Midlife Hand Grip Strength as a Predictor of Old Age Disability"
> Journal of the American Medical Association
> 1999;281:558-560.

Stress—The Builder/Destroyer—and Yoga

The term stress—the state of being where one is outside one's comfort zone—is applied to both living and inanimate objects. Mechanical and civil engineers talk of stress limits beyond which engine parts fail and bridges collapse. Stress is also important in developing strength—even in the inanimate world. The blacksmith hammers the red hot iron bar to create powerful tools. Without this hammering and heat the metal tools would just break apart. For the human body, stress is needed to develop sharp minds and strong bodies. Without intellectual challenges how will a child's mental abilities grow? And without subjecting our muscles to stress through play and exercise we will have flabby, weak bodies. Stress, real or perceived, can also destroy the body and mind. On a purely physical level stress beyond a certain point can cause tears in the muscles and cause serious injuries.

While excess physical stress can be avoided by a well planned and executed exercise and work program, mental stress is more insidious. A perception of real or imagined danger, a threat, loss of control, or betrayal triggers a flood of neural responses. Neurotransmitter chemicals, especially norepinephrine (or noradrenaline) appear and create heightened focus, awareness, and anxiety. These chemicals are necessary for our survival. The fight-or-flight response is critical for us. Being in this state for long periods, however, causes premature aging and loss of connection with reality.

The impact of mental stress on premature aging can be understood through the cell biology process of cell duplication, death, and mutation. Our body (and that of all living creatures) is made up of cells that are continually duplicating themselves and dying. The duplication process is mediated by our DNA so that exact copies of the cell are made. However, once in a while there is a mutation in the cell and an incorrect copy is made of the cell. Some of these mutations simply die out and the duplication process just stops. Other times some mutated cells (especially cancer cells) can duplicate endlessly, essentially killing the human body.

Stress creates the chemical changes in our body that appear to be conducive to both death of cells and the mutation of cells. The stress can be directly physical in cases such as smoking, ingesting carcinogenic chemicals, living in polluted areas, and absorbing excess radiation from the sun,. etc. But the stress can also be mental where perception alone can cause chemical conditions responsible for premature aging and disease.

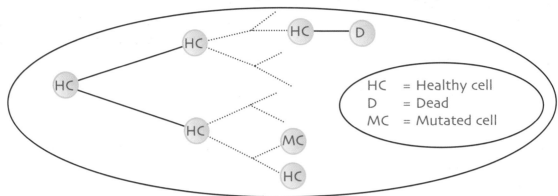

The key ingredients of yoga—calmness, breathwork, mental awareness of the body, muscles pushed outside the comfort zone—are together capable of breaking the feedback loop created by mental stress. The RussaYog session with its added bal-lila (child's play) prepares the mind and body for joy, fun, and optimism that is then locked in by the asans and breathwork.

It is well known that drugs—legal and illegal—can also lift the shadow of excessive stress and provide relief from the negative symptoms of mental stress. But drugs come with negative side effects—some quite serious. Of course, for severe cases, drug intervention may be appropriate. However, by following a consistent, holistic approach such as RussaYog, one arms oneself with an important tool to help handle the negative effects of stress.

Easing Disease

Among the prosperous of the world the dominant diseases are heart disease, stroke, hypertension, and diabetes. Additional irritants that lower the quality of life are back problems, arthritis, sexual dysfunction, fatigue, sleep disorders, and digestive and breathing problems. While genetics play a role in many of these diseases, a significant source of these illnesses is lifestyle choices. Many studies have shown the role that "bad stress" (high-fat/high-calorie diet, sedentary lifestyle, lack of proper breathing, and lack of exercise) contributes to poor health.

YOGA AND DISEASE

A yoga-based exercise program and lifestyle is fast emerging as an important tool in physical (and mental) well-being. It is our belief that the RussaYog practice described here can be a powerful way of improving one's sense of well being. In particular the following connections can be made between various elements of RussaYog and improved health:

BREATHWORK: The slow, deep breathing exercises, especially performed while the body is under stress, enhances lung capacity and improve oxygen uptake. Greater oxygen flow should help energize the body and help reduce fatigue.

FLEXIBILITY: Bal-lila helps blood flow and greatly improves flexibility. A key sign of old age is loss of flexibility—not entirely due to any organic process, but also due to lack of use. Bal-lila does not involve any bouncing or pounding movements, yet raises the heart rate to an aerobic level.

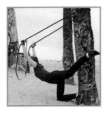

HEART HEALTH: Bal-lila increases the heart rate, thereby strengthening the heart muscle.
Veer-lila, with little rest, is an excellent way to raise the heart rate. Breathwork teaches the student to stay calm and use stress to build and grow, not panic.

DIABETES: Asans in which flexibility is increased by bending backward are suggested for diabetes. Bridge Asan, Agni Lapat, and Ulta Kaam Asans accomplish this.

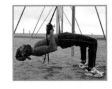

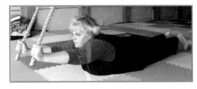

BACK PROBLEMS:
Ek, Doh, and Teen Dharat Namaskar and Bal-lila help strengthen the lower back, especially while consciously engaging the abdominal muscles.

RESTLESSNESS: The use of Drishti, Pranayama, and Asans helps one learn to focus.

PULMONARY PROBLEMS: Deep breathing. Inhale-Exhale-Hold the breath while compressing the abdominal muscles.

FATIGUE: Deep breathing exercises and shoulder stand.

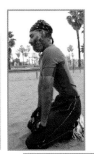

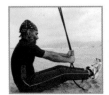

SEXUAL HEALTH:
All four Kaam Asans develop strength and enhance blood flow into our core.

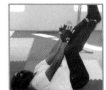

ARTHRITIS OF KNEES AND JOINTS:
Jhoola Asan and Agni Lapat each help strengthen supportive muscles.

The overall RussaYog session can also place the yogi into an efficient, yet unhurried state which is essential for healthful living.

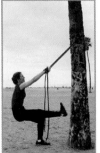

Some Questions with Answers

• Can RussaYog help me lose weight?
Weight loss has emerged as one of the most important physical and psychological health issues in "rich" societies. While complex social, psychological, and evolutionary issues control the desire to eat, once the food is in your body, four parameters control weight loss or gain:

> 1. Caloric intake from food
> 2. Efficiency of converting food to "body"
> 3. Metabolism, i.e, rate of caloric use per unit of work done
> 4. Energy expended through exercise and daily work.

RussaYog, like traditional yoga, is a calming exercise. It forces one to maintain balance under forces pulling from different directions. It allows the practitioner to learn how to maintain balance and a mental vision of "detached-attachment." Such a balance should allow one to modify the first parameter listed above (caloric intake). This is critical for weight loss. Just slowing down the eating process can greatly influence how much food one eats. An hour of RussaYog burns about 300 Calories. The resultant muscle growth also helps by burning calories faster.

The human body is incredibly efficient—a single candy bar can allow a typical human to walk about 2 miles. So it is difficult to lose weight just through exercise.

• How is RussaYog different from traditional yoga?

On the physical level traditional yoga places the body in asans (or poses) which test the body's flexibility. In some asans the practitioner also needs great balance and (usually) lower body strength. The asan is then held for anywhere from 10 seconds to several minutes, or, in a few cases, hours. In some forms of traditional yoga, accessories like belts, chairs, blocks, etc., are added.

The RussaYog session takes the mind through all four states of shant, chanchal, sthir, and supt. In particular it takes the yogi through the chanchal (playful) state. In traditional yoga this state is not addressed. The use of mudra (physical, mental, and emotional preparation) and vishram (rest, stretch) provide bookends to each asan in RussaYog. This is generally not done in traditional yoga practices. Additionally, focus on chardi kala (unbounded optimism) is unique to RussaYog yoga.

In RussaYog a free flowing rope, looped over an anchor in the ceiling (or a tree branch or a playground swingset...) is gripped. This allows the user to manipulate the direction of the force of gravity. The RussaYog practitioner can do asans that would otherwise require one or several "helpers." The practitioner of RussaYog can not only develop flexibility and balance, but also strength and stamina normally associated with weight training.

• How does RussaYog compare to weight training?

Weight training is based on using movable weights (either directly or through machines, such as pulleys) to stress muscles and thus strengthen them. Weight training is an excellent exercise to build strength and, if done correctly, posture. Over the last several decades there has been an intense effort made by equipment designers to take weight training away from "free weights" to large machine-based workouts. The benefit of this trend (apart from profits for equipment makers) has been that many more people, some with injuries or weaknesses that would not allow them to work out with free weights, can participate. The downside to this trend is that the user does not have to depend upon "balance" and the use of many core muscles. Weight training can also cause an imbalanced body appearance (disproportionately huge upper body, compared to small leg muscles, etc.).

RussaYog provides the muscle strength available through weight training, although one cannot build huge muscles, since one uses the body's own weight for resistance. It is particularly good for core muscles and balance. It also "lifts" the body frame for an erect posture. Most importantly, in RussaYog the asan is held for several breaths and the focus is on a mental-physical connection.

137

unbounded optimism ॐ हिन्दी

• How does RussaYog influence the aging process?

Most people are already familiar with changes brought on by aging, like thinning of hair, loss of hair color, diminution of memory, and decreasing sense of balance. The vexatious characteristics of cynicism and mental rigidity can also be casualties of aging. In the U.S.A. (and many other developed countries) the aging process is also character-ized by the following (statistical based) changes:

> • An increase in weight of 1 to 2 pounds per year from ages 25 to sixty. This is accompanied by a loss of about 1% of muscle strength per year from age 25.
> • A combination of unhealthy diet and work habits causes weakening abdominal muscles making the abdomen sag outward—even for thin people.
> • A gravity-driven drooping of the shoulders, breasts, and buttocks, and a lowering of erection angle for men appears to go hand in hand with sagging abdominal muscles.

It would be incorrect to say that a practitioner of RussaYog will not age! However, the counter-gravity use of ropes and strengthening of core trunk muscles can postpone or even banish the first three aging-related processes. A number of RussaYog asans pull the body up and "gently backward"—as if a physical therapist was working with you.

• Can anyone do RussaYog?

Anyone can do some parts of RussaYog. However, since many asans require a strong grip, strong upper body, and trunk strength, practitioners should slowly build up to them. Athletes who are already participating in sports (runners, swimmers, football players, rowers, etc.) should have no problem doing the full offering of asans. A good rule of thumb for anyone would be the following:

Can you grip a bar and hold your body hanging off the ground for 5-10 seconds? If you cannot, it is good to do an easier version of the asans shown.

Certainly if you' have had back, shoulder, knee, or wrist surgery, please check with your physician before starting. Modify your hold if you feel any pain, or simply avoid the asan. Push yourself beyond your comfort zone, but never at the cost of pain or injury.

• Does RussaYog improve sexual abilities?

While sex involves complex physical and psychological issues, there is no question that the physical part is closely tied to physical fitness. An important part of erectile dys-function is related to high cholesterol, obesity, and high blood pressure. After all, male erection and female arousal have to do with good blood flow.

The lingam-yoni asans (i.e., the Kaam asans) of RussaYog are especially useful for developing the groin and abdominal muscles, the core muscles. This sequence of asans should help the physical aspect of sexual fitness.

1

• How does yoga in general and RussaYog in particular contribute to spiritual health? Let us first define a general concept of our spiritual being—a sense that we are part of a bigger picture. The phrase "Ik Onkar" or "one source, many manifestations" summarizes a spiritual view of the Universe. You are spiritual if you can extend beyond the "me-versus-you" duality. Yoga does not automatically make you spiritual. However, the calming nature of yoga can help quiet the mind and look at the Universe with a "big picture" view—to simultaneously see our infinitesimal and infinite form. The RussaYogi learns to keep a calm balance, enhancing one's abilities to improve as a spiritual being.

• What kind of body "look" does RussaYog create?
Many fitness programs are indeed associated with a certain kind of appearance: the strong, but gaunt look of distance runners; the powerful look of sprinters; the heavily muscled look of body builders, etc. Based on the kind of asans in RussaYog and the muscles they stress a practitioner should expect to develop the lean, strong look of trapeze artists. RussaYog also balances the body so deep core muscles which may not be "show muscles" are developed.

• Should I take any special precautions while doing RussaYog?
It is important, as in any demanding exercise program, to warm up. A special warm up and strengthening procedure has been designed for RussaYog. Additionally, it may be useful to wear gloves (for example, weight-training gloves) so that the pressure of the ropes does not cause discomfort. After a few sessions the hands and wrists will strengthen, but it is a good idea to use gloves or any other hand wrap (like those used by gymnasts) to protect the hands and fingers. If you feel stiffness in the fingers, do fewer movements that place undue stress on your fingers and combine the rope-based movements with non-rope-based movements shown in this book. Occassionally you may feel finger stiffness in the morning if you have been doing intensive training. Opening and closing the fingers will help reduce the stiffness. Your hands will get accustomed to gripping. Grip strength is a good indicator of overall health. (see refernce on page 133)

• Will RussaYog make me feel good while I'm doing it and after?
Absolutely! Most students feel a sense of elation during and after the asan. The combination of quick, powerful movements and the calm holding asans releases a burst of endorphins. Many students feel a sense of optimism and a "pump" resulting from enhanced blood flow. Not only does RussaYog produce a balanced mind and body—the process itself is a pleasure. You should see benefits even if you do the full RussaYog session once per week.

• Sometimes my mind is locked into negative thoughts. Can RussaYog help me get out of these states?
To escape negative thoughts (assuming one is not in need of medical treatment for depression) one needs to enter the chanchal state. This requires playful activity. The Bal-Lila portion of the RussaYog session is excellent for this.

• How can RussaYog asans and workout be integrated with other workouts for a highly fit physique?

Our experience with our studio members is that a twice-a-week RussaYog session (one hour each) is quite adequate for developing a balanced core. For optimum health a person should exercise an hour per day. You may do the full RussaYog session (60 minutes) twice a week, and the other days use some elements of RussaYog with other exercises. For example, on days you do not do a RussaYog session you may still practice pranayam for five minutes and incorporate some aspects of bal-lila into your workout. In addition, you may choose to walk, run, swim, weight train, or any other sport activity you enjoy.

Bibliography

Ornish, Dean, M.D., "Dr. Dean Ornish's Program for Reversing Heart Disease: The Only System Scientifically Proven to Reverse Heart Disease Without Drugs or Surgery" New York, Ballantine Books (1996).

Sparrowe, Linda and Walden, Patricia, "Yoga for Healthy Bones: A Woman's Guide," Shambhala Publications, Inc., Boston, MA (2004).

A number of excellent web resources now exist for people to use. These include the Mayo Clinic website and the National Institute of Health website.

Why Punjabi?

The yoga asans and their accompanying emotional and physical states are described in Punjabi. Punjabi, the 11th most spoken language, is an amalgam of Sanskrit, Hindi, and numerous loaner words form Persian, Urdu, English, Dutch, and dialects of other Indian languages. It is the language of Chardi Kala, where small things are treated as major events. A friend is greeted as a Brave Warrior, a customer is greeted as King of the Universe, a child is called a Lion or Lioness. A piece of bread is called mouth-watering cake.

Punjabi is spoken in Northern India and in Pakistan, and Punjabis are settled all over the world. Much of the Guru Granth Sahib is written in a form of Punjabi. It is the language of Bhangra, the dance for the young at heart. It seems to me that while traditional yoga asans are described in Sanskrit, the power and behavior of RussaYog asans should be described in Punjabi.

The great intrigues of Mahabharat were enacted in the land of the Punjab (now split into the Indian states of Punjab and Haryana). This is where Lord Krishna imparted the Bhagvad Gita to Arjun, laying the foundation of yoga.

Here are some common terms which capture the essence of Punjabi spirit

ਚੜਦੀ ਕਲਾ	Chardi kala	used in response to "how are you?"
ਬਲੇ ਬਲੇ	Baley, baley	everything is coming up roses
ਵੀਰ, ਵੀਰੇ	Veer, Veerey	warrior (for brother, friend)
ਸਜਨ	Sajan,	dear friend
ਮਹਾਰਾਜ	Maharaj	can be used for anyone on the street
ਜਲ ਛਕੋ	Jal Chhuko	have this delicious nectar (a glass of water)
ਚਕ ਦੇ	Chuk de	just do it!
ਪਰਸ਼ਾਦੇ	Prashad	term for simple bread, but means a delicious meal
ਪ੍ਰੇਮਿਯੋ	Premiyo	my lovers (used for friends, family, strangers)
ਭਗਤੋ	Bhagato	saints (used for friends/strangers)
ਮੇਰੇ ਮੀਤ	Merey meet	my friend
ਜਾਨੇ ਮਨ	Janey man	dearer than life (friends or even strangers)
ਸ਼ੇਰਾ	Shera	lion, lioness
ਫੋਜਾਂ	Faujah	means "army," but used for one or two friends

RussaYog tries to imbue the yogi with the spirit of Chardi kala where

    a cool glass of water tastes like exotic nectar
    a hug from a friend is like a restful night in a palace
    a piece of bread shared with a lover is like a feast at a 5-star restaurant
    a beautiful sunrise is like a trip to the Louvre
    a child's laughter is like a visit to La Scala Opera House
    (250 to 450 Euros/seat for 2007)
    a swing on a rope is like a night with an Arabian Houris
    (or the equivalent male Arabian stud)
    a moonlit walk with a close friend is like a visit to the Taj Mahal
    an effortless teen dharat namaskar is like a massage
    an agni lapat asan is like a visit to Cirque du Soleil

Feast of Words (glossary)

ਚੜ੍ਹਦੀ ਕਲਾ *unbounded optimism*

Aadhaar, Foundation
Aashram, Place to learn yoga
Abhay, Fearless
Abyas, Exercises
Agni, Fire
Akal, Timeless
Anand, Bliss
Anhad, Without boundaries
Antar, Inside
Arjun, Archetypal ideal warrior
Asan(a), Yoga pose
Ashtanga, Eight branches
Ath, Eight
Avastha, State

Baal, Child
Bahar, Outside
Bal, Strength
Bal-lila, Child's play
Balvan, Powerful
Bhagvad Gita, Hindu holy text
Bhangra, Vigorous folk dance
Bharosa, Trust
Bhav, Attitude
Bhog, Fruits of Karma
Brahmin, Caste (highest),
  Learned person
Bund, Closed

Chakar(a), Circles
Chanchal, Playful
Char, Four
Chardi kala, Unbounded
  optimism
Chey, Six

Dand, Punishment
Dus, Ten
Dhanwadi, Grateful
Dharat, Earth
Dhyan(a), Attentive mind
Doh, Two
Drishti, sight

Ek, One
Ekta, Oneness, harmony

Garabh-lila, Birth drama
Garurh, Eagle
Gurdwara, Sikh place of worship

Gur Parsad, Guru's Blessings
Guru, Teacher
Guru Granth Sahib, Holy
  book and final Guru for
  the Sikhs
Gurumukhi, Punjabi script

Halasan, Plough pose
Hath, Hand
Hukam, Law

IkOnkar, One source

Jaag, Awake,
Jaagya, Awakened
Jag, Universe
Jhoola, Swing

Karma, Action
Kichh, Pull
Khul, Open
Khoj, Exploration
Kirit, Earnings through
  effort
Kirtan, Devotional singing
Kriya, Action
Kundalini, Hidden energy

Lachak, Flexibility
Lapat, Flame
Lila, Drama
Lingam, Male sex organs
Lord Krishna, Hindu incarnation

Mahabharat, Indian pic
Man, Mind
Mantra, Words to meditate on
Mooldhara, Root chakra
Mudra, Preparatory gesture

Namaskar, Humble
  salutation
Nauw, Nine
Nihal, Bliss
Nirala, Unique
Nirvair, Without prejudice
Nirvan(a), Merge into infinte
Nishchey, Resolve
Nischint, Worry free
Niyama, Disciplined living

Panj, Five
Parvat, Mountain peak
Prakriti, Nature
Pran, Life
Pranayam(a), Breathwork
Pratyachara, Inward eye

Russa, Rope
RussaYog, Rope yoga

Saat, Seven
Sadhu, Person who has
  withdrawn from society
Samadhi, Merge into infinite
Sarbat ka bhala, All flourishing
Sat Nam, True word
Sehej, Balance
Shabad, Enlightened word
Shakti, Power
Shant, Calm
Shavsan(a), Corpse pose
Shiatsu, Japanese massage system
Sikh, Person of Sikh faith, student
Simran, Meditation
Sthir, Focused
Sundar, Beautiful
Supt, Rest

Tadasan(a), Mountain pose
Teen (tin), Three
Trikonasan(a), Triangle pose
Tulsi, Herb, holy basil

Ulta, Up-side down

Veer, Warrior
Veer-lila, Warrior drama
Vishram, Rest
Vishram Beach, RussaYog
  Retreat locale
VishramYog, RussaYog-style
  massage
Vishvaas, Confidence

Wah, Wonder

Yama, Practice
Yatra, journey
Yog(a), Union
Yogi, Person who seriously
  practices yoga
Yoni, female sex organs

Ode to russa (rope)
Pliable, powerful, purposeful.
Pleasure-giver to chldren.
Sailors and adventurers love you.
You make us feel young!

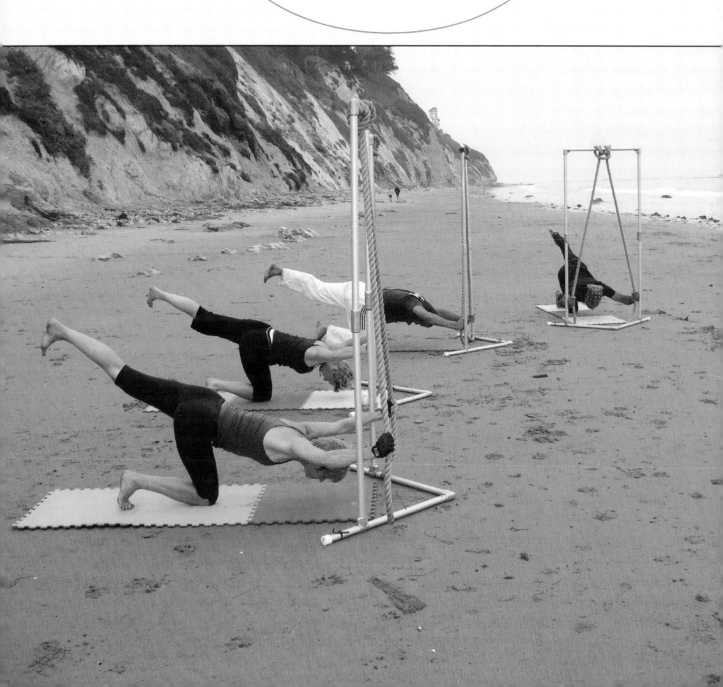

Training, Certification, and Tools of the Trade

Having gone through this book you already feel energized by the simplicity and power of RussaYog. How do you begin? RussaYog is an easy, holistic fitness program that can be learned through the following paths:

- Contact us to see if there is a certified teacher in your area.
- Obtain one of our DVDs that will take you through the session. Ask for the DVD that best suits your needs.
- Consider attending one of our retreats.

You may be able to find an anchor from which to hang the rope. Or you can purchase our portable, light-weight RussaYog Primal Shakti Yoga Tree, which offers you the flexibility of doing RussaYog wherever you want.

Ask your health club, yoga studio, or martial arts studio if their instructors can get certified to teach RussaYog.

TOOLS OF THE TRADE

Rope, one-inch thick jute
Gloves (weight training or bicycle gloves will do)
One or two yoga mats, or 3, 6, or 9 interlocking mats
An anchor for the rope.

Fixed anchor: Beams in a studio, chin-up bar, tree branch in a park, palm tree on the beach, or play structure with a high (8 foot) bar.

Portable structure: Primal Shakti® Yoga Tree I and II.

Self-study: RussaYog instructional DVDs.

PRIMAL SHAKTI YOGA TREE I	PRIMAL SHAKTI YOGA TREE II

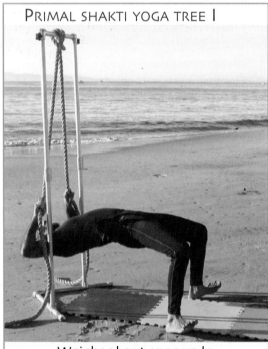 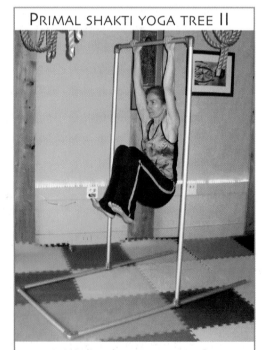

Weighs about 15 pounds.
Can be carried in a small bag.
Suitable for athletic students.

Weighs about 20 pounds.
Suitable for low-mobility users,
since it offers more stability.

Contact us at talk@russayog.com
Visit us at www.russayog.com

Teacher Training

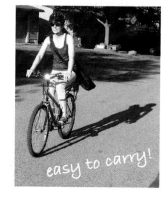

(personal trainers, yoga instructors, fitness clubs, martial arts and dance studios)

Share your joy: Become a certified RussaYog instructor!

Once you experience the joy of RussaYog Primal Shakti® workouts you will want to share this experience with others.

Becoming a RussaYog instructor is easy! Are you:

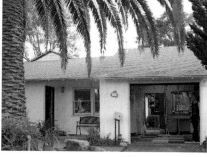

- a trained yoga instructor (private practice, studio, or gym)
- a personal trainer (private practice or gym)
- martial arts teacher (tae kwon do, karate, aikido, etc.)
- dance teacher
- physical therapist (private practice/health care)
- fitness center owner/manager with instructors

easy to carry!

A 200-hour training (at home and under our supervision) can get you trained as a RussaYog instructor. The training covers:

Physical aspect: Pranayam, bal-lila, veer-lila, nirvan, and how-to of Yoga Tree and studio setup. Also elements of shiatsu—passive yoga, vishram massage.

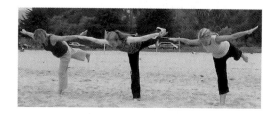

Philosophical aspect: Achieving coherence in our physical body, achieving coherence in body and mind, in me-and-society and in me-and-Universe.

Karmic wealth concept: How to understand and enhance karmic wealth, which includes valued wealth (dollars), relationship wealth (friends), catalytic wealth (barrier-lowering wealth), and sacred (life-affirming) wealth.

Financial aspect: How to teach part-time/full-time and succeed.

Contact us at talk@russayog.com

vishram beach ashram in California

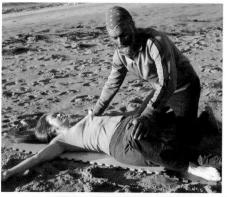

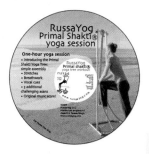

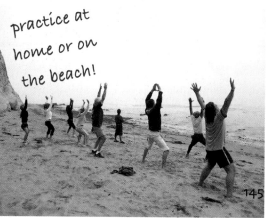

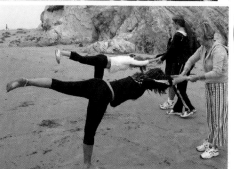

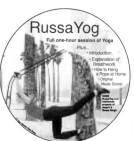

practice at home or on the beach!

145

Retreaters enjoying morning pranayam on the beach during a RussaYog retreat at Vishram Beach Aashram in Santa Barbara, California.

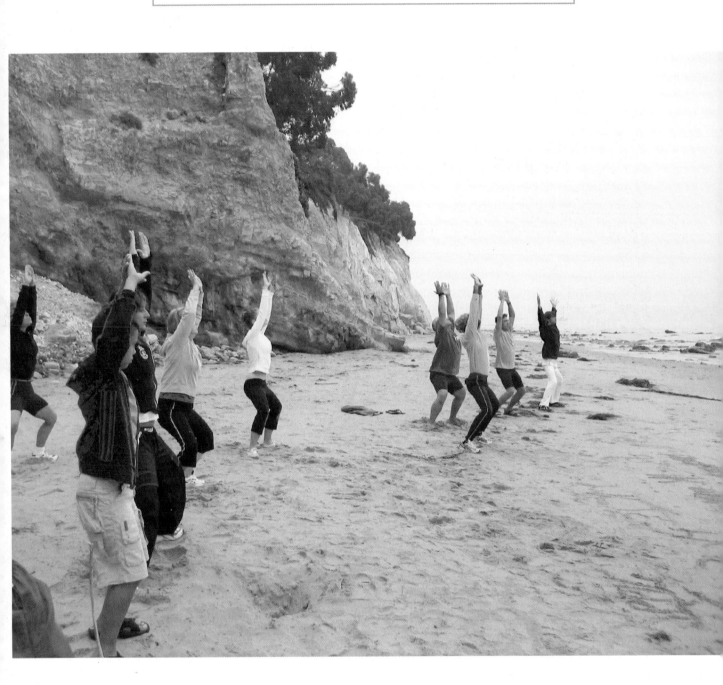

RussaYog Asan Sequence

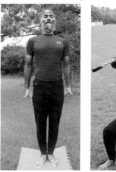
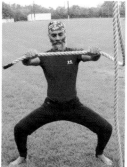

Tadasan · Russa Kichh

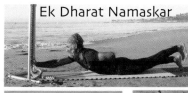
Ek Dharat Namaskar

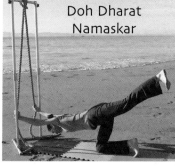
Triconasan on knees · Baalasan

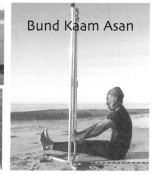
Bund Kaam Asan

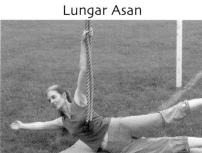
Lungar Asan

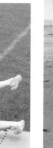

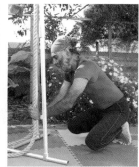
Doh Dharat Namaskar

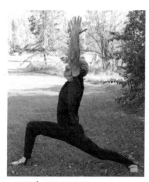
Balasan Press on Knees

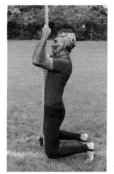
Balasan Pull on Knees

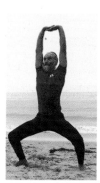
Parvat Asan

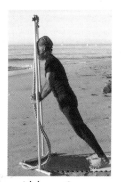
Abhay Asan

Ek Veer Asan

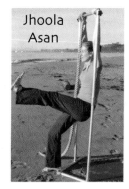
Jhoola Asan

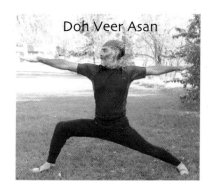
Doh Veer Asan

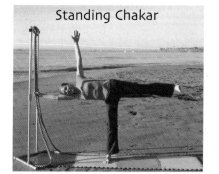
Standing Chakar

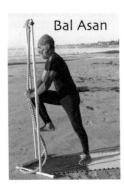

Bal Asan

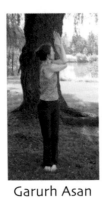

Teen Dharat Namaskar

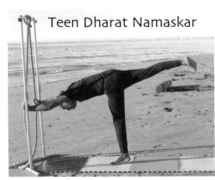

Arm Stretch

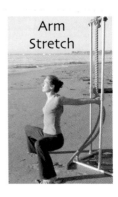

Garurh Asan

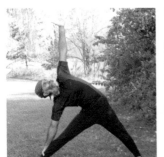

Triconasan

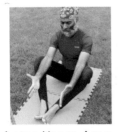

Ek Veer Asan with Ropes

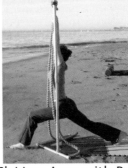

Savaar Asan

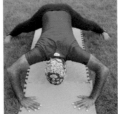

Seated Twist

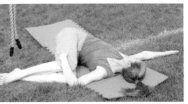

Ulta Antar Kaam Asan

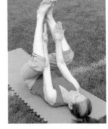

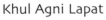

Antar Kaam Asan

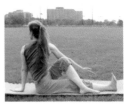

Jag Namaskar III

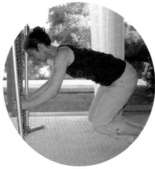

Bridge Asan

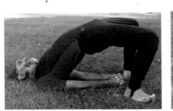

Lying Down Twist

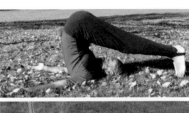

Khul Agni Lapat

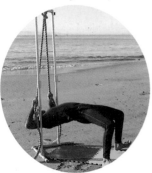

Dand Agni Lapat

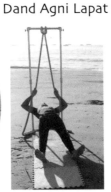

Shoulder Stand

Halsan

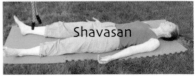

Shavasan

148 copyright ©2007 Jasprit & Teresa Singh